Total
Quality and
Productivity
Management in
Health Care Organizations

Total Quality and Productivity Management in Health Care Organizations

Vincent K. Omachonu

American Society for Quality Control
Milwaukee, Wisconsin

Industrial Engineering and Management Press
Institute of Industrial Engineers
Norcross, Georgia

Published by the Institute of Industrial Engineers and the American Society for Quality Control.

Figures 1-6 and 1-7 are reprinted with permission from *AHA Hospital Statistics,* copyright 1989 by the American Hospital Association.

Figure 9-2 is reprinted with permission from *AHA Hospital Statistics,* copyright 1987 by the American Hospital Association.

Printed in the United States of America.

95   94 93   92   91   5   4   3   2   1

Library of Congress Cataloging-in-Publication Data
Omachonu, Vincent K.
Total quality and productivity management in health care organizations / Vincent K. Omachonu.
p.   cm.
Includes bibliographical references and index.
ISBN 0-89806-113-X
1. Hospitals--Administration.   I. Title.
[DNLM: 1. Health Facilities--organization & administration--United States.   2. Quality of Health Care--United States.   W 84 AA1 05t]
RA971.045   1991
362.1'1'068--dc20
DNLM/DLC
for Library of Congress   91-21753
CIP

Quantity discounts available from:
Publication Sales
Institute of Industrial Engineers
25 Technology Park
Norcross, Georgia 30092 USA

Contents

List of Acronyms

AHA - American Hospital Association
ANA - American Nurses' Association
DRG - Diagnosis Related Group
FTE - Full Time Equivalent
JCAHO - Joint Commission on Accreditation of Healthcare Organizations
LOS - Length of Stay
LPN - Licensed Practical Nurse
MFPMM - Multi-factory Productivity Measurement Model
MIS - Management Information System
PDCA - Plan/Do/Check/Act
PPS - Prospective Pricing System
PR - Provider-Receiver
PRO - Peer Review Organization
QA - Quality Assurance
QC - Quality Control
QFD - Quality Function Deployment
QIRA - Quality in Routine Activities
RN - Registered Nurse
TARP - Technical Assistance Programs, Inc.
TQC - Total Quality Control
TQM - Total Quality Management
TSQC - Total Service Quality Control
TSQM - Total Service Quality Management

Foreword

There is good news and bad news in the ever changing health-care industry. If health-care administrators do not create statements of vision and mission, develop strategic and short term plans, identify key performance indicators and optimum practice levels, the government will step in and do it for them. The tools, knowledge, and mindset required to begin this transformation are available and attainable through Total Quality Management (TQM).

To ensure a bright and promising future TQM must replace the engineering management models of the past. Dr. Omachonu's book provides excellent insight into the theory and practice of TQM as it relates to the health-care industry. A clear road map for the transition of old management styles in the health-care industry to the new management and engineering paradigms of TQM can be found within the pages of this book.

Howard S. Gitlow
Coral Gables, Florida

Preface

Never before in the health-care industry has there been such intense emphasis and open debate on the issues of quality. The steady rise in the cost of health care coupled with the need for quality and competitiveness have combined to put the health-care industry at the top of the national agenda for reform.

The days of unlimited consumption of health-care resources are over, as competitive pressures force many health-care organizations to close their doors or streamline operations. The health-care industry is experiencing tremendous pressure to reform. The needed change calls for a new philosophy and operational paradigm. The transformation must be deliberate and focused; it must seek to identify quality and cost containment as complementary rather than antagonistic objectives. The transformation should not be based only on a definition of quality from the Joint Commission on Accreditation of Healthcare Organizations (formerly the Joint Commission on Accreditation of Hospitals). It should also be driven by the customer's needs and wants. What is needed today is a visible affirmation of top management's commitment to pursue quality as an important mission of the organization.

Quality is not just a socially provocative idea. Quality and cost are two of the most important criterion by which people evaluate their health-care purchasing decisions. Quality has become a key strategic level for health-care management in the face of a growing number of highly informed consumers. A health-care organization that is not keeping its eyes on the customers, external and internal, is slowly endorsing a prescription for failure. Today's health-care organizational culture is driven by the notion that management and/or the provider knows best. The truth is that the customer knows best and should be a part of the process and service design.

One of the initial challenges for health-care managers lies in understanding how improved quality can ultimately lead to increased productivity. This book explains the relationship between quality and productivity, and shows how quality leads to competitiveness and long term survival.

This book is unique in both content and approach. It discusses quality and productivity and shows how to achieve them. Dozens of examples and illustrations of the tools needed to realize quality and productivity are provided.

The quality concepts discussed in the book are driven by the philosophies of Dr. W. Edwards Deming and Drs. K. Ishikawa, S. Mizuno, and Asaka. This book presents total quality management (TQM) in the context of three critical and interconnected components—quality, productivity, and technology management. Throughout the book, the link among all the three components is preserved.

Health-care executives, managers, supervisors, middle managers, management engineers and professionals (e.g. physicians, nurses, pharmacists, and therapists) will benefit from this book. The needs of students in health administration are also addressed.

Acknowledgements

This book is the result of several years of work in the area of service quality, productivity, and technology management. Several people have helped to shape my views on quality, productivity, and technology management in health care, and it would be impossible to name them all here. I remain eternally grateful to them for supporting my interests and pointing me in the right direction. Special thanks to Professor Ravinder Nanda of the Polytechnic University in Brooklyn, New York for helping me take my first step into the health-care field. Thanks also go to the University of Miami Institute for the Study of Quality for providing the proper environment to develop my research interests, and to the Department of Industrial Engineering, University of Miami, for the opportunity to write this book.

I also wish to thank the various health-care organizations and their staff who provided the data and information used in this book. Their insights are reflected in the material presented in this book.

My sincere gratitude goes to the various manuscript reviewers whose invaluable suggestions and comments brought this book to its present form.

Finally, I wish to thank my wife Abo, my daughter Amanda, and my son David, for their patience and understanding of my need to write this book. While this book does not do everything that it could do, I hope that in some small way, it serves as a guiding light for individuals in the health-care field who wish to walk the long dark path to quality. And most of all, my deepest gratitude to God for making it all possible.

Miami, Florida
1991

Vincent Kema Omachonu

xv

Part One

Foundations of Quality and Productivity

This section presents the underlying foundations of quality and productivity issues in health-care organizations. Chapter One discusses the quality and cost challenges facing health-care organizations by presenting some of the hard realities facing the industry. The relationship among the three critical components in the book (continuous quality improvement, productivity, and technology) is established, as well as the connection with Dr. W. Edwards Deming's chain reaction. Cost breakdown is presented at the micro and macro levels, in addition to how cost constraints affect the present health-care environment.

Chapter Two analyzes the basic definitions of productivity and quality in health care, followed by a discussion on various proposed methodologies for understanding costs. This material provides an essential background against which the rest of the book rests.

The material presented in this section is vital to any meaningful effort towards the management of quality and productivity in health-care organizations. The effective management of total quality and productivity must be preceded by a clear understanding of the intervening factors affecting today's health-care environment.

1 The Challenges Facing Health-Care Organizations

This book takes an integrated approach to the management of quality, drawing upon the interrelationships between quality and productivity, and between quality and technology. A graphic representation of this interrelationship is presented in Figure 1-1. Many experts agree that quality improvement leads to productivity increases. This relationship is not fully understood in health-care organizations, however. Major misconceptions that quality can only be achieved through huge capital investments in elaborate and sophisticated technologies continue to exist among American health-care managers. Health-care administrators are often misled into spending huge sums of money without first giving a chance to small but continuous improvements. It amounts to a policy of buying "quality" through costly technology-related strides in improvement, as opposed to small but steady, more cost efficient, and deliberate improvement efforts involving all employees.

The old paradigm is based on the notion that quality means CT Scanner or Magnetic Resonance Imagers (MRI) technologies. The concept of continuous improvement strategy for quality implies that quality is a process rather than an outcome.

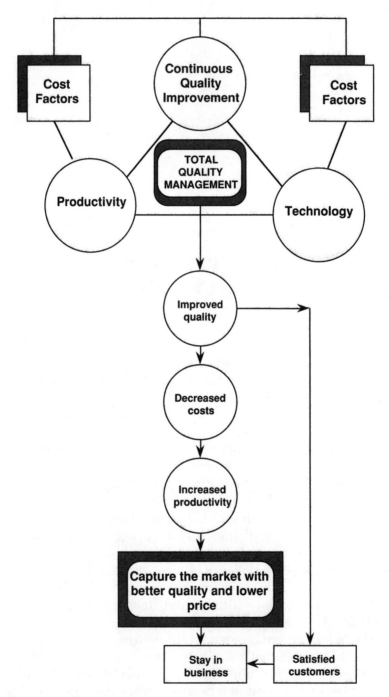

Figure 1-1. Total quality management triangle.

Technology can be used to support quality and productivity through the use of information systems. The challenge facing management information systems in health care is one of supporting productivity and quality efforts by generating reliable and adequate information. If quality improvement is pursued only through technology, then increased quality may decrease productivity. According to Dr. Deming's (1986) chain reaction, improved quality leads to decreased costs, and increased productivity, both of which enhance an organization's ability to capture the market, stay in business, and have satisfied customers. Consequently, it is imperative to fully understand the concepts of costs, productivity, and technology, as vital components of quality.

UNDERSTANDING THE HEALTH-CARE BUSINESS

Health-care expenditures have experienced a rapid growth from $42 billion (5.9 percent of the Gross National Product or GNP) in 1965 to nearly $700 billion (12 percent of GNP) in 1990. It is projected that health care should account for almost 20 percent of GNP by the year 2000 (Dressler 1990). Figure 1-2 shows the growth in health-care expenditures as a percentage of GNP.

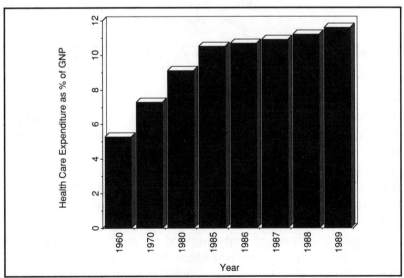

Figure 1-2. Health-care expenditures as a percent of GNP. *(Source: Health Care Financing Review, 11(4) and 12(2).)*

Health-care expenditures in 1988 were $497 billion. The largest percentage of dollars—39 percent—was spent on hospital care. Figure 1-3 shows a breakdown of U.S. health-care dollars for 1988.

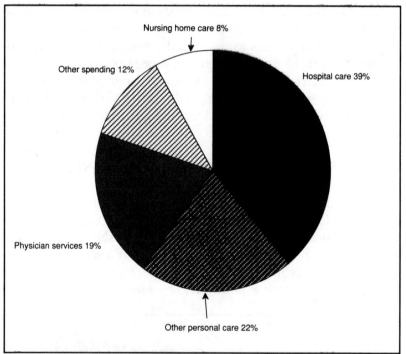

Figure 1-3. Distribution of health-care expenditures in 1988. *(Source: Health Care Financing Review, 11(4).)*

In order to understand health-care costs, it is essential to understand the sources of health-care spending as depicted for 1988 in Figure 1-4. Similar figures for long-term care are presented in Figure 1-5.

As mentioned previously, the largest percentage of expenditures in 1988 was for hospital care (see Figure 1-3). A further breakdown of the expenses incurred by hospitals for the same year is shown in Figure 1-6.

These figures show that the need for cost containment has never been more compelling. Many hospitals are closing their doors due to rising health-care costs and the inability to effectively contain costs and manage quality. For example, fifty

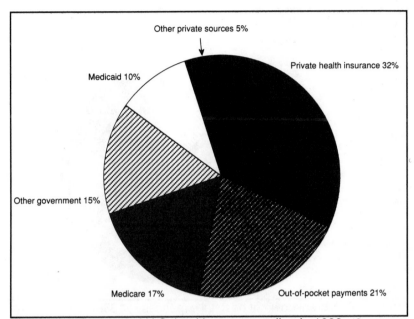

Figure 1-4. Sources of U.S. health-care spending in 1988. *(Source: Health Care Financing Review, 11(4).)*

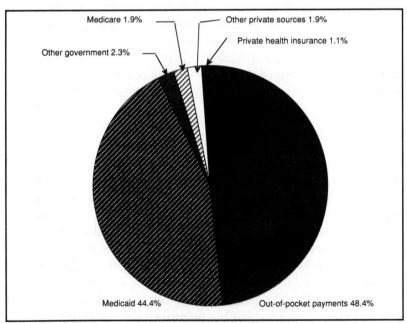

Figure 1-5. Sources of U.S. long-term care payment in 1988. *(Source: Health Care Financing Review, 11(4).)*

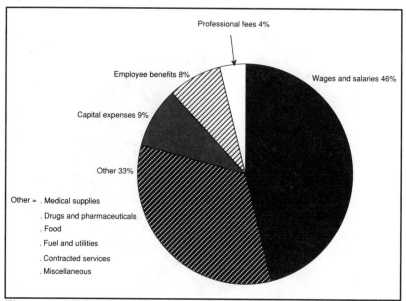

Figure 1-6. A breakdown of hospital expenses in 1988. *(Source: AHA Hospital Statistics.)*

percent of all U.S. hospitals currently lose money treating Medicare patients (McCarthy 1988). In certain cases, hospitals received no more than 72 cents on the dollar for services provided to Medicaid patients and about 89 cents on the dollar for medicare patients. Figure 1-7 shows the frequency of urban and rural hospital closures in the U.S. between 1980 and 1987.

THE SERVICE INDUSTRY

The health-care industry and other service industries differ from the manufacturing and processing industries in many ways. There are many similarities, however. The typical hospital specializes in a wide range of complex services that must be provided day and night, seven days a week. Like other businesses, the hospital must compete for land, labor, capital, and entrepreneurial ability. And, like manufacturing organizations, it is also expected to pass the profitability test.

In essence, then, a hospital is a business—in fact, by any measure, one of the largest businesses in the United States. To illustrate this further, a summary of the similarities and differ-

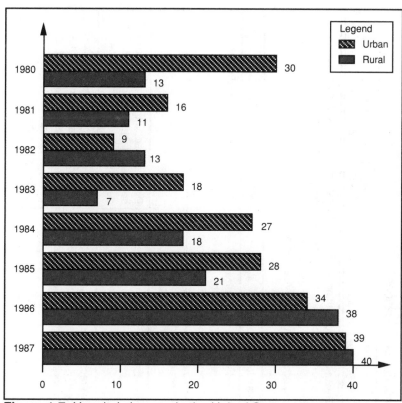

Figure 1-7. Hospital closures in the United States. *(Source: AHA Hospital Statistics.)*

ences between the service and manufacturing sectors and the place of hospitals in the overall picture is presented in Table 1-1. Health care is a unique industry, yet certain aspects lend themselves to management techniques used in manufacturing and other service industries.

TODAY'S HEALTH-CARE ENVIRONMENT

The health-care field today finds itself in an environment in which its services must be viewed as vital components of some 490 "product lines" known as Diagnosis Related Groups (DRGs). The idea of equating services to product lines represents a business orientation and is often unattractive to many in the health-care profession. The previous system of reimbursement

Table 1-1. Characteristics of manufacturing versus service organizations.

Factor	Manufacturing Product Systems	Service Product Systems	Using Hospital Nursing Unit as an Example
Product (output)	Physical creation of goods. Transformation of input into a tangible physical product.	Treatment of something or someone. Processing of knowledge and skill into a product that is not physical in nature. Service implies an act.	Patients (diversity of diagnosis implies multiple products).
Labor	Less labor intensive.	More labor intensive.	More labor intensive.
Mechanization	Higher mechanization generates products with low variability. Smooth and more efficient. Task is repetitive. Physical products often lend themselves to a considerable amount of standardization.	Low degree of mechanization. Greater output variability. Task is mainly non-repetitive. Outputs do not lend themselves to standardization.	Mainly non-repetitive tasks. Every patient is different.
Customer contact	Low customer contact. Allows separation of production and consumption.	High degree of customer contact.	Direct contact with recipients of services. Health-care cannot be delivered prior to arrival of patients.
Quality control	Allow for recalls, warranties, scrap, and rework.	No recalls, warranties, scrap, rework, etc. Use of damage control to appease a dissatisfied customer.	Ongoing quality assurance programs. Quality standards must include patients' perception of quality. Huge possibility of malpractice suits.

Factor	Manufacturing Product Systems	Service Product Systems	Using Hospital Nursing Unit as an Example
Product (output)	Physical creation of goods. Transformation of input into a tangible physical product.	Treatment of something or someone. Processing of knowledge and skill into a product that is not physical in nature. Service implies an act.	Patients (diversity of diagnosis implies multiple products).
Labor	Less labor intensive.	More labor intensive.	More labor intensive.
Mechanization	Higher mechanization generates products with low variability. Smooth and more efficient. Task is repetitive. Physical products often lend themselves to a considerable amount of standardization.	Low degree of mechanization. Greater output variability. Task is mainly non-repetitive. Outputs do not lend themselves to standardization.	Mainly non-repetitive tasks. Every patient is different.
Customer contact	Low customer contact. Allows separation of production and consumption.	High degree of customer contact.	Direct contact with recipients of services. Health-care cannot be delivered prior to arrival of patients.
Quality control	Allow for recalls, warranties, scrap, and rework.	No recalls, warranties, scrap, rework, etc. Use of damage control to appease a dissatisfied customer.	Ongoing quality assurance programs. Quality standards must include patients' perception of quality. Huge possibility of malpractice suits.

can be characterized as one of "cost maximization," in which no ceilings were placed on the amount of money that hospitals were allowed to charge for their services. Reimbursement was determined primarily on the basis of the costs incurred in providing patient care. Under the present reimbursement system known as Prospective Pricing System (PPS), hospitals are reimbursed a fixed amount for a given patient DRG, irrespective of costs.

As a result, members of the health-care profession are challenged to pursue the dual objectives of ensuring an acceptable quality of care in a fiscally restrained environment. Health care is a humanistic profession whose academic and professional preparation emphasize the need to provide the best quality care based on human need. Those who have been trained in the old school of thought find some of their professional values challenged in today's environment of cost containment. Traditionally, the emphasis has been on saving lives, not dollars.

Impact of DRGs

To gain an understanding of the benefits of the prospective pricing system, it is helpful to know the problems associated with the previous reimbursement approach used by hospitals to determine costs for health-care services provided to patients (Davies et al. 1983). The previous reimbursement approaches:

- encouraged the use of patient day as a unit of service for establishing cost and reimbursement.
- did not provide true incentives for health-care providers to contain costs.
- tended to have regulations focused on hospitals even though they are merely suppliers of treatments ordered by physicians.
- did not apply to all payers but rather to some defined subset of major payers.
- defined cost in a manner that did not cover the full financial elements of the hospital.
- generally lacked comparability of costs, given that institutional comparisons are used to determine cost norms.
- employed peer-grouping methods based on self-predicting

variables that tended to institutionalize the cost behavior of high-cost providers.
• lacked sensitivity and fairness with respect to case-mix differences.

The benefits of tying the costs of services to DRGs are many. Zeigenfuss (1985) describes the following:

• some control is offered over rising health-care costs
• hospitals are challenged to provide quality care within the new, reduced health-care expenditure limits
• doctors benefit by streamlining their treatment so that optimum care is provided consistent with limited health-care resources
• diagnoses, for reimbursement purposes, are improved and scrutiny is increased (also care quality is increased as a result of improved diagnoses)
• a large and sophisticated data base for research, service improvement, cost monitoring, and training is developed
• action is taken on the cost problem, which increases sensitivity to costs and raises awareness of the need for change
• a further linkage of clinical and managerial action is provided which strengthens the hospital organization as a whole

The DRG system is not without negative impact, however. Some of the negative impacts, concerns, and effects associated with the DRG system are as follows (Zeigenfuss 1985, Howard 1984):

• hospitals have gone out of business
• many decisions are now being made by the managers of the system, as opposed to clinicians and direct care providers
• access to the health-care system is limited
• the system creates a business mentality incompatible with the rendering of good, quality care
• DRGs depersonalize medical care
• patients do not fit into neat categories
• some are "good" DRGs and are usually promoted, while others are shortchanged
• medical malpractice has risen tremendously

Incentives to decrease services provided to patients are a by-product of DRGs. The decrease in level and quality of services provided may be viewed as a "rational" response to the constraints of DRGs (Schwartz 1983).

Additional effects of DRGs are as follows (Lave 1984):

- Length of stay for a particular diagnosis has decreased. The use of home health agencies, nursing-home beds, and rehabilitation centers have increased.

- The number of admissions and readmissions in many cases has increased. Some patients who could be treated as outpatients are being treated as inpatients. In addition, there is incentive to space treatments or operations (if possible) rather than to do them during the same hospital episode. This incentive is even stronger for those hospitals experiencing decreased occupancy rates—induced in part by the shorter lengths of stay encouraged by PPS.

- Some illegitimate diagnosis recording takes place. For example, a DRG with a higher reimbursement may sometimes be substituted for one with a lower reimbursement (when the lower reimbursement DRG is the primary DRG).

- Some providers may attempt to "skim" patients within a given DRG; that is, they may try to select only the relatively inexpensive patients within a given DRG and transfer the patients with more serious conditions elsewhere.

- Services that have been cross-subsidized by other services are likely to be phased out. Some of the services—such as social services, nutritional counseling, health promotion, or prevention activities—may be services that contribute to a decrease in the cost of post-hospital care, but to an increase in inpatient costs.

Summary

In today's DRG environment, one need not look very far to observe that most of the predicted impacts of DRGs are indeed accurate. What is perhaps most obvious is the fact that hospitals which ignore costs and quality simply cannot survive. While hospitals do not have control over revenues generated per DRG, they still have a significant control over the resources consumed in the delivery of care. The real challenge in the decade of the 1990s is how to pursue the objectives of quality health care in a fiscally restrained environment. The issue is by no means trivial.

EXERCISES

1-1. Present a pie chart similar to Figure 1-5, showing the breakdown of your hospital's expenses for the current year. How do the figures compare to the ones presented in Figure 1-5?

1-2. Develop a study to determine the amount of money your hospital received on the dollar for services provided to Medicaid and Medicare patients during the past five years. What conclusions can you draw from the figures? What percentage of your revenues is due to Medicaid and Medicare?

1-3. What are some of the negative impacts of DRGs on your institution? What are the positive impacts? How have the costs of medical malpractice changed since the introduction of DRGs?

BIBLIOGRAPHY

Davies, R. H., G. Westfal, et al. 1983. Reimbursement under DRGs: Implementation in New Jersey. *Health Services Research.* 18(2):233-244.

Deming, W. E. 1986. *Out of Crises.* Cambridge: MIT CAES.

Dressler, G. 1990. As health care expenditures grow so does the potential for jobs. *Miami Herald Business Monday.* July 30:43.

Howard, R. B. 1984. DRGs prospective payment/prospective horror. *Postgraduate Medicine.* 76(1):13-14.

Lave, J. E. 1984. Hospital reimbursement under Medicare. *Milbank Memorial Fund Quarterly.* 62(2):251-268.

McCarthy, C. M. 1988. AHA president quoted by Linda Oberman. *AHA News.* September 12.

Omachonu, V. K. and R. Nanda. 1988. A conceptual framework for hospital nursing unit productivity measurement. *Industrial Engineering.* Norcross, GA: Institute of Industrial Engineers. 20(5):56.

Schwartz, W. 1983. The competitive strategy: Will it affect the quality of care? *Market Reform in Health Care.* J. A. Meyer, ed. Washington, DC: American Enterprise Institute.

Sorrentino, E.M. 1989. Hospitals vary by LOS, charges, reimbursements and death rates. *Nursing Management.* 20(1):54.

Ziegenfuss, Jr., J. T. 1985. *DRGs and Hospital Impact.* New York: McGraw Hill Book Company.

2 Productivity, Costs, and Quality Issues in Health Care

The term "productivity" as applied to health care has been defined in several different ways depending on who is defining it—nursing professionals, health economists, hospital administrators, management engineers, etc. Several different measurement approaches have been proposed for studying the subject, including quality assurance. Part of the problem is that the "product" is ill-defined and highly varied. There continues to be disagreement among health-care professionals as to what constitutes the output of a health-care facility.

DEFINITIONS OF PRODUCTIVITY

Productivity is defined generally as the ratio of output to input. Health-care researchers and practitioners have offered a diverse range of definitions from the perspectives of nursing, nursing units, DRGs, patient outcome, etc. While most of these definitions raise important questions, few offer any practical guidelines toward implementation.

DiVesta (1984) notes that nursing productivity is strongly associated with the costs of delivering care. When services are delivered inefficiently, the costs in most cases are higher and the effectiveness of the service is lessened. There are some in the health-care field who feel that hospital productivity can only be fully defined in the context of nursing productivity. Dennis and Jelinek (1976) define nursing productivity as "the amount and quality of output produced for a given amount of input." Output is defined in terms of number of nursing hours available. Curtin and Zurlage (1986) define nursing productivity as "the relationship between inputs and outputs." Levine (1984) defines nursing productivity as "the ratio of nursing services required (output) to the amount of nursing hours actually expended, modified by a quality factor (input)." Other literature sources define nursing productivity as the ratio of work output to work input (Gray and Steffy 1983, Haas 1984, and Ganong and Ganong 1984). Management consultants have also made their marks in defining nursing productivity. In a conference report put out by the participants in the National Invitational Conference on Nursing Productivity (1986), the following observations were made regarding management consultants:

> ...a flood of management consultants market software to nursing administrators to define productivity as nursing hours per patient day or hours per workload index....Only if nurses continue to buy these definitions, both literally and figuratively, will these vendors continue to thrive.

In 1974, Jelinek, et al. conducted a survey in the Medicus Corporation that culminated in the definition of nursing productivity and the development of a model to assess it. The definition of nursing productivity in this project began with its traditional definition: the relationship between the amount of acceptable output and input required to achieve the desired output. Operationally, the definition became the ratio of the intensity of nursing care required on a nursing unit to the equivalent amount of registered nursing hours available to provide patient care, modified by the quality of nursing care provided. The quality of nursing care was determined by the quality scores from the Rush-Medicus quality assessment approach.

Curtin and Zurlage (1986) discuss nursing productivity in terms of outcomes. They describe outcomes as the sum of the inputs made where the "system" meets the consumer. Curtin and Zurlage note that, "For health services, productivity lies in the surplus values added in the course of access, attendance, treatment, education, rehabilitation, and follow-up. Measurement begins with the assessment of input status at T_1 of both the served (physical and emotional status, personal characteristics, etc.) and the server (resources available, server status at T_1, etc.). Measurement takes place in terms of negotiated outcomes for both the served and the server at T_2."

A three-part economic-based definition of nursing unit productivity was developed by Omachonu and Nanda (1988) as follows:

1. Total Productivity of a Nursing Unit. The total productivity of a nursing unit is defined as the ratio of the output to input of the unit, where output is stated in terms of the total DRG revenues generated by all patients admitted in the unit (and for whom nursing care was provided), and input is stated as the costs of all resources consumed (direct nursing care, indirect nursing care, room and bed, fixed and variable overhead, and ancillary costs). Both input and output are adjusted to base-period prices (constant dollar terms). When a quality factor is used as a multiplier to this model, it yields the quality-adjusted total productivity of a nursing unit.

2. Productivity of Nursing in a Given Unit. The productivity of nursing in a given unit is defined as the ratio of output to input with respect to nursing. Output is stated as the portion of the total DRG revenues attributable to nursing intervention. This is achieved by multiplying the total DRG revenue values by an adjustment factor given as a ratio of the hospital nursing cost (direct and indirect care) to total cost of the hospital. Input is stated as the direct and indirect cost of nursing care. Both input and output are adjusted to base-period prices.

3. Productivity of Individual Diagnosis. Diagnosis-based productivity is defined as the ratio of diagnosis-based output to diagnosis-based input. Diagnosis-based output is stated as the total DRG revenues generated by patients treated for a given diagnosis during the productivity measurement period. Input is the cost of the resources consumed in treating patients of the specific DRG. Some inputs cannot be entirely traced to a given DRG; they are adjusted by a factor that is given as the ratio of total patient days in that DRG to the overall patient days in the unit. Both input and output are adjusted to base-period prices.

COST CONSIDERATIONS

It is generally believed that physicians have the primary responsibility for controlling costs in health care, since they determine what kinds of services a patient needs and how much of it. There are other costs, however, that neither physicians nor other health-care practitioners directly control (Donabedian 1988). Donabedian explains as follows:

> For example, if as a result of overbuilding or unskillful scheduling, hospitals remain partially empty, the cost of care goes up and so does the cost of improving health, without health-care practitioners being necessarily at fault.

Nursing care costs also represent a huge portion of total health-care costs. Caterinicchio and Davies (1983) measure nursing resource use in a way which permits the allocation of nursing costs on a per case basis by discharge diagnosis. This involves the determination of the hours of care consumed by patients. Walker (1983) and Riley and Schaefers (1984) use a patient classification system to measure nursing care costs. According to Riley and Schaefers, the total nursing cost is given as the sum of direct nursing costs, nursing unit costs, and nursing administration costs respectively.

In their study, Riley and Schaefers conceptualize nursing costs in two different ways—direct nursing costs and total nursing costs. Direct nursing costs are those associated with all aspects of nursing care provided to a patient based on intensity. This includes all aspects of assessing, planning, implementing, and evaluating nursing care. Total nursing costs are defined as all direct costs plus the costs of nursing unit support personnel, nursing supervision, in-service education, and nursing administration. Riley and Schaefers note that "while direct costs reflect all aspects of individual care, total nursing costs reflect resources necessary to provide a nursing super-structure to create an environment in which to provide nursing care." For example, orientation and in-service education programs are certainly legitimate nursing costs. All patients should bear a portion of the expense regardless of whether the patients benefitted directly from these programs.

According to Nunamaker (1983), Medicare's efficiency measure consists of multiple inputs (e.g., direct nursing hours, supplies, allocated overhead, etc.) aggregated by price (cost) weights, and the total divided by an equally weighted measure of outputs (patient days). In their work on nursing resources, Mitchell, Miller, Welches, and Walker (1984) translate into costs the total hours of nursing care for admission in the following way. The hours of care given are multiplied by the average hourly salary and benefits for direct care given on the respective units. The correct percentage of each care giver on the unit is used to determine the average salary for the unit. Also, Sovie, et al. (1984) utilizes a patient classification system as a basis for assessing the cost of patient care.

Omachonu and Nanda (1988) suggest that the nursing unit is the most suitable point to study resource consumption for inpatients. The resource input of a nursing unit is divided into two categories: nursing care costs and non-nursing care costs. The complete breakdown is presented in Chapter Five.

QUALITY OF CARE CONSIDERATIONS

Competition for patients among hospitals has forced the health-care industry to take a strong look at the quality of care provided to patients. Before the 1930s, there was seldom any consideration given to the quality of our nation's health care. Since then, widespread interest in the relationship between quality and health care has been generated. Many views on the basis for good medical care and how to measure quality are available. For example, in 1914 Codman presented views about improving the quality of products of a hospital by evaluating the end results of treatment. Lee and Jones (1933) presented a comprehensive view of what constitutes "good medical care." Donabedian (1966) presented what is today a universal classification of quality according to structure, process, or outcome. Outcome refers to the consequence or benefit of medical intervention. Process refers to the activities of physicians and others involved in the care of patients. Structure examines the qualifications, certifications, and similar attributes of the resources used in care delivery. According to Donabedian (1980), defining quality of care requires a definition of the attributes of the care as well as criteria for what constitutes good care. Wyzewianski (1988) notes:

> Traditionally hospitals have competed for patients only indirectly. The focus has been on attracting and retaining physicians, who in turn bring in patients. To lure physicians, the bait has often been the availability of better facilities and equipment and greater responsiveness to individual physician preferences. In the new era of surplus hospital beds and surplus physicians, however, patients are courted more directly.

Apart from huge investments in advertisement, there is a tremendous emphasis on friendly and courteous personnel as well as attractive facilities.

Donabedian (1980) points out that the activities involved in the management of illness can be divided into two domains: the technical and the *interpersonal*. Donabedian has defined technical care as "the application of the science and technology of medicine, and of the other health sciences, to the management of a personal health problem." The interpersonal aspects of care involve the social and psychological aspects of the health-care professional-patient interaction. Donabedian has also referred to a third aspect of care which is the *amenities* of care. The amenities of care refer to the elements of comfort, convenience, and attractiveness of facilities.

Cleary and McNeil (1988) note that what is frequently overlooked is that patients can play an important role in defining what constitutes quality care by determining what values should be associated with different outcomes. Ginsburg and Hammons (1988) explain, "Care is of good quality insofar as it contributes to the patient's health and well being." Quality has also been linked to patient satisfaction. Pascoe (1983) defines patient care as a health-care recipient's reaction to the salient aspects of their service experience.

As the debate continues over what quality means to whom, increasing attention is being paid to the relationship between quality and outcome. In their work on quality assurance, Luke, Krueger, and Modrow (1983) describe the principle of quality assurance by stating that "the hospital shall demonstrate a consistent endeavor to deliver patient care that is optimal with available resources and consistent with achievable goals." Several measurement instruments have been developed for the purpose of assessing quality of patient care and also for comparing the performance of nurses providing care to patients. Egdahl and Gertman (1976) point out that in the last 60 years, nearly 1,000 studies have been performed to assess the level of quality of care delivered. These studies use a variety of data collection techniques—from direct physician observation to claims form review. They examine either structural, process, or outcome variables. Virtually all of these studies detect basic problems in the level of quality of care delivered.

OUTCOME MEASURES

One classic list of outcome measures (Lohr 1988) comprises "the five Ds": death, disease, disability, discomfort, and dissatisfaction. Death, especially when it is unexpected, premature, untimely, or avoidable, is often taken as an indicator that quality of care may have been compromised (Lohr 1988). The use of death as an outcome measure, and the prospect of using avoidable death as a useful and valid outcome indicator have been widely studied (Blumberg 1986; Dubois, Brook, and Rogers 1987; Carr-Hill, Hardman, and Russell 1987; and Eggers 1987). The prospects of using death as an indicator of outcome raises several questions:

• Can or should such measures be used to draw conclusions about quality of care or only to serve as screens, because they do not appear to be particularly useful in deciding what to do in situations where quality seems deficient?

• Can mortality measures be extended to reflect physician-specific monitoring?

• Should post-hospitalization deaths be included, and to what extent?

• What are the effects of severity of illness, case mix, sex, age, and prior hospitalization on mortality rates?

• If it is possible to adequately adjust for severity and case mix, would there be enough information and variability across institutions to make mortality rates reliable indicators of quality?

• What are the effects on mortality rate of factors such as socioeconomic class, race, nutritional condition, family support, and attitudes towards medical care?

According to Donabedian (1980), outcomes are indicators of quality of care only if they are attributable to process and structural elements, rather than being the result of genetic, environmental, or other factors.

Wyszewianski (1988) makes the following observations concerning outcomes:

> The almost reflexive response to the current desire for simple, understandable measures of quality—measures that can both inform and reassure a suddenly uneasy public—has been to turn to outcome measures such as hospital mortality rates, while more or less openly disparaging structure and process measures.

Curtin and Zurlage (1986) describe the outcomes of nursing practice as the promotion, enhancement, or restoration of persons to their optimal state of functional competence. Curtin and Zurlage remark:

For individual members of the public, outcome expectations are conditioned by degree of general education and opinion (political, social, and commercial), and lifestyle. For professionals, negotiated outcome expectations are expressed in terms of practice standards and norms. For the community, acceptable outcomes are expressed in terms of statutes, regulations and case law. For health institutions, expected outcomes are seen in terms of income, community reputation, and market share. Finally, for payers, outcome expectations are seen in terms of contractual obligations expressed in dollar limits, time limits, and review of the care regimen.

The degree of uncertainty and debate about these issues is high. Until they are resolved, caution in the aggressive application of mortality rates as outcome measures is warranted (Lohr 1988). Other forms of outcome measures often mentioned include readmission to hospitals and reoperations (perhaps secondary to unanticipated surgical complications).

The Joint Commission on Accreditation of Healthcare Organizations has responded to the growing concern of underprovision of care due to DRG-based reimbursement by embarking on a historic shift towards outcome measures (O'Leary 1987).

A change in emphasis to outcome measures implies a results-oriented program, which can be very destructive. The concept of TQM is based on a process orientation. To define quality in terms of outcome assumes that the process is under control and predictable. Outcome measures also imply that the employee is responsible for results rather than management.

SUMMARY

Quality, productivity, cost, and outcome are among the many complex issues facing health-care administrators. Quality should be defined in terms of conformance to standards as well as the needs and wants of the customers. Productivity should be driven by the total resources consumed in the delivery of care. In order to fully understand productivity, we must first understand all cost components. Although outcome is important, it is even more important to understand that the process generates the outcome.

EXERCISES

2-1. What definitions of productivity do you use at your facility? How do they differ from the ones presented in the chapter?

2-2. Discuss the advantages and disadvantages of outcome measures.

2-3. What performance indicators do you use in place of formal productivity measures?

2-4. What is quality in health care?

BIBLIOGRAPHY

Berwick, D. M. and M. Knapp. 1987. Theory and practice for measuring health care quality. *Health Care Financing Review.* (ann. suppl.) 9:49-55.

Blumberg, M. S. 1986. Risk adjusting health care outcomes: A methodological review. *Medical Care Review.* 43:351-393.

Brook, R. H. 1973. Quality of care. *Journal of Medical Education.* 48:114-134.

Brook, R. H. and K. Lohr. 1985. Efficiency, effectiveness, variations, and quality: Boundary crossing research. *Medical Care.* 23:710-722.

Brook, R. H., K. Williams, and A. Avery. 1976. Quality assurance today and tomorrow: Forecast for the future. *Annals of Internal Medicine.* 85:809-817.

Carr-Hill, R. A., G. Hardman, and I. Russell. 1987. Variations in avoidable mortality and variations in health care resources. *Lancet.* (April 4):789-792.

Caterinicchio, R. and R. Davies. 1983. Developing a client focused resource use: An alternative to the patient day. *Social Science and Medicine.* 17:259-272.

Cleary, P. D. and B. McNeil. 1988. Patient satisfaction as an indicator of quality care. *Inquiry.* 25:25-36.

Codman, E. A. 1914. The product of a hospital. *Surgery, Gynecology and Obstetrics.* 18:491-496.

Curtin, L. L. and C. Zurlage. 1986. Nursing productivity: From data to definition. *Nursing Management.* 17(6):32.

Dennis, L. C. and R. Jelinek. 1976. A review and evaluation of nursing productivity. *Health Manpower References.* (DHEW) Pub. no. (HRA) 77:15.

Divesta, N. 1984. The changing health care system: An overview. *DRGs: Changes and Challenges.* F. A. Shaffer, ed. New York: National League for Nursing. Pub. no. 20.

Donabedian, A. 1966. Evaluating the quality of medical care. *Milbank Memorial Fund Quarterly: Health and Society.* 44:166-206.

_____. 1980. *The Definition of Quality and Approaches to Its Assessment.* Ann Arbor, MI: Health Administration Press. p. 27.

_____. 1985. Twenty years of research on the quality of medical care, 1965 - 1984. *Evaluation and the Health Professions.* 8:243-265.

_____. 1988. Quality and cost: Choices and responsibilities. *Inquiry.* 25:90-99.

Dubois, R. W., R. Brook, and W. Rogers. 1987. Adjusted hospital death rates: A potential screen for quality of medical care. *American Journal of Public Health.* 77:1162-1167.

Egdahl, R. and P. Gertman. 1976. *Quality Assurances in Health Care.* Gaithersburg, MD: Aspen Systems Corporation.

Eggers, P. W. 1987. Prospective payment system and quality: Early results and research strategy. *Health Care Financing Review* (ann. suppl.).

Elinson, J. 1987. Advances in health assessment conference discussion panel. Donabedian, et al. *Journal of Chronic Disease.* 40, suppl. 1:183s-191s.

Ganong, J. M. and W. Ganong. 1984. *Performance Appraisal for Productivity: The Nurse Manager's Handbook.* Rockville, MD: Aspen Systems Corp.

Ginsburg, P. B. and G. Hammons. 1988. Competition and the quality of care: The importance of information. *Inquiry.* 25:108-115.

Gray, S. P. and W. Steffy. 1983. *Hospital Cost Containment Through Productivity Management.* New York: Van Nostrand Reinhold Co.

Haas, S. W. 1984. Sorting out nursing productivity. *Nursing Management.* 15(4):37-40.

Jelinek, R. C., R. Haussmann, S. Hegyvary, and J. Newman. 1974. *A Methodology for Monitoring Quality of Nursing Care.* DJEW Washington, DC: Government Printing Office. (January) Pub. no. (HRA) 76-25.

Levine. 1984. Some issues in nursing productivity. *Costing Out Nursing: Pricing Our Product.* Franklin A. Shaffer, ed. New York: National League for Nursing. Pub. no. 20-1982. p. 237.

Lohr, K. N. 1988. Outcome measurement: Concepts and questions. *Inquiry.* 25:37.

Luke, R. D., J. Krueger, and R. Modrow. 1983. *Organization and Change in Health Care Quality Assurance.* Rockville, MD: Aspen Systems Corp.

Mitchell, M., J. Miller, J. Welches and D. Walker. 1984. Determining cost of direct nursing care using DRGs. *Nursing Management.* 15(4).

Nadler, G. and V. Sahney. 1969. A descriptive model of nursing care. *American Journal of Nursing.* 69:336-341.

National Invitational Conference on Nursing Productivity Conference Report. 1986. Georgetown University. October.

Nunamaker, T. R. 1983. Measuring routine nursing service efficiency: A comparison of cost per patient day and data development analysis models. *Health Services Research.* 18(2).

O'Leary, D. 1987. The Joint Commission looks to the future. *Journal of the American Medical Association.* 258:951-952.

Omachonu, V. K. and R. Nanda. 1988. Hospital nursing unit productivity measurement: A conceptual framework. *Industrial Engineering.* Norcross, GA: Institute of Industrial Engineers. 20(5):56.

_____. 1989. Measuring productivity: outcome vs. output. *Nursing Management.* 20(4):35.

Omachonu, V. K. 1990. Quality of care and the patient: New criteria for evaluation. *Health Care Management Review.* 15(4):43.

Pascoe, G. C. 1983. Patient satisfaction in primary health care: A literature review and analysis. *Evaluation and Program Planning.* 6:185-210.

Phaneuf, M. 1973. Quality assurance: A nursing view. *Hospitals.* p. 62.

Riley, W. J. and V. Schaefer. 1984. Nursing operations as a profit center. *Nursing Management.* 15(4):43.

Sorrentino, E. M. 1989. Hospitals vary by LOS charges, reimbursements and death rates by DRG category. *Nursing Management*. 20(1):54-60.

Sovie, M. D., M. Tarcinale, A. Van Putte, and A. Stunden. 1984. A correlation study of nursing patient classification, DRGs, other significant patient variables and costs of patient care. *Final*. (November).

Wyszewianski, L. 1988. Quality of care: Past achievements and future challenges. *Inquiry*. 25:13-22.

Part Two

The Management of Health-Care Quality

This section discusses the concept of health-care service quality management from the perspective of the customer. The theme of this section is that quality should be defined in the context of the customer's experiences, needs, and wants.

Chapter Three presents a detailed discussion on quality as perceived by the customer as well as the critical factors that influence the customer's perception. Other important issues discussed include patient expectations, an understanding of who the customers are, and a discussion of the quality of provider behavior.

Chapter Four begins with a discussion of the major quality theories that have shaped our thinking during the past four decades. These theories are examined in the context of the health-care environment. The application of Dr. Deming's 14 points to health care is also presented in Chapter Four. The bulk of Chapter Four deals with the application of the seven Quality Control (QC) tools for the continuous improvement of total quality. Both inpatient and outpatient case examples are presented throughout the chapter. Later in the chapter, the concept of Quality Function Deployment (QFD) is discussed, with applications in health care. The chapter concludes with a road map for the implementation of Total Quality Management (TQM) in health-care organizations.

3 Understanding Health-Care Service Quality

Today's health-care environment is continuously changing. It is being constantly challenged to respond to consumers' growing demands for good and acceptable quality of care. Perhaps a necessary starting point lies in your organization's response to the following key question:

WHAT DOES QUALITY IN HEALTH CARE MEAN IN YOUR ORGANIZATION?

- Meeting the requirements of the Joint Commission on Accreditation of Health Care Organizations (JCAHO)
- Doing your best for your customers
- Meeting or exceeding the expectations of health-care customers
- All of the above

Today's health-care customer has a distinct list of expectations. Hospitals that make a conscious effort to respond to these expectations are certain to emerge as the leaders among health-care organizations in the 1990s. Perhaps the critical test of how well a hospital meets or exceeds the expectations of its consumers may be found in the answers to the following four questions:

Patients:

1. Would you enthusiastically recommend this hospital to someone you love?

2. If you have a say in the matter, would you come back to this hospital for treatment?

Health-care professionals:

3. Should you need medical treatment, would you (as a physician, nurse, or other clinical professional) make this hospital your first choice?

4. Would you (as a physician, nurse, or other clinical professional) select this hospital as your place of practice?

If a hospital cannot obtain "yes" answers to these questions, then it should reexamine its commitment to quality. Responses such as "maybe," "perhaps," and "possibly" are simply not good enough. Such responses only falsely reinforce an already fragile commitment to quality. One of the goals must be to obtain a "yes" response to each question. While a "yes" response may not be the absolute test for good quality, it could mean an initial indicator of some level of commitment.

QUALITY OF CARE AND THE CUSTOMER: NEW CRITERIA FOR EVALUATION

For many years, hospitals have (through agencies such as JCAHO) dictated what is "good" for the patient and sometimes how much of this "good" the patient is entitled to. Little or no attempt was made towards finding out the patient's perception of quality. The JCAHO (1990) defines the quality of patient care as follows:

The degree to which patient care services increase the probability of desired patient outcomes and reduce the probability of undesired outcomes, given the current state of knowledge.

In today's health-care environment and in other service organizations, JCAHO's definition of quality would be considered inadequate and misguided in that it fails to address an essential component—the patient's viewpoint. Quality as perceived by the recipient of care is critical to the complete definition of quality. The definition by JCAHO is also deficient because it focuses on the present not the future, and because it is results oriented instead of process oriented.

Quality consists of two interdependent parts: quality in fact and quality in perception. The first involves meeting your own specifications (conformance to standards), and the second part is meeting the expectations of your customer. Neither of these in itself will carry a hospital far. To deliver health care exactly as JCAHO intends will be to no avail if potential patients believe you are providing inferior service. Also the quality of the services provided by the support functions, such as accounting or billing, does not necessarily improve because of your adherence to the requirements of JCAHO.

Quality of Conformance

Two major organizations responsible for providing guidelines for health-care quality standards are The American Nurses' Association (ANA) and JCAHO. These two organizations, together with state licensing agencies, also set standards for nursing care.

The JCAHO accredits about 83% of the nation's community hospitals. Its stamp of approval allows hospitals to be government certified. Medicare patients account for about 40% of an average hospital's revenue (Millenson 1987). Also, the federal government employs private, non-profit groups called Peer Review Organizations (PROs) to keep an eye on hospital's quality.

In the early 1960s, Donabedian developed a framework that discussed quality in terms of three factors: structure, process, and outcome. Quality of structure meant a hospital was clean, safe, and had all the right equipment in its operating rooms and patient areas. Process quality meant that the medical staff used the equipment correctly. Outcome meant that the patient got well—or at least did not become worse any sooner than he or she would have without the medical staff's intervention. Donabedian (1980) says that he sees process and outcome as complementary. In the mid-1970s, the JCAHO began requiring hospitals to perform process and outcome reviews in addition to structure reviews.

Quality Monitoring at the Nursing Unit Level

In general, a quality monitoring methodology (quality assurance) defines the nursing process as the comprehensive set of nursing activities performed in delivering a patient's care. This overall process is carried out in three phases as follows: assessing the needs of the patient, planning for care, and updating the plan of care by evaluating the patient's response to the current care plan. By considering assessment, planning, and evaluation, this tool is said to measure nurses' performance beyond technical functioning.

It is critical to note that there are major differences between the Quality Assurance (QA) approach to quality and the Total Quality Management (TQM) approach to quality. Some of the differences are outlined below:

• Quality Assurance is driven by standards prescribed by the JCAHO, whereas TQM puts every employee in the organization in charge of quality.

• Quality Assurance stresses conformance to standards (quality in fact), whereas TQM stresses quality in fact and quality in perception.

• Quality Assurance assumes that the JCAHO knows best and should dictate what good quality means, whereas TQM is driven by a definition of quality based on the needs, wants, and expectations of the customers.

• Quality Assurance in some organizations means preparation for an announced visit from the JCAHO, by staging a show to reflect good quality assurance, whereas, TQM is a never-ending activity of continuous improvement.

- An on-going QA activity involves a group of in-house professionals who make sporadic visits to the units to check for compliance and identify problem areas, whereas, TQM involves everyone in the organization (telephone operators, receptionists, secretaries, nurses, unit support staff, medical records clerks, etc).

- Most QA activities are driven by episodic measurements. Data gathering is usually carried out in response to an episode or a crises, whereas, TQM emphasizes the need to focus on the process generating the episodes and to put mechanisms in place to better control the process.

- Quality assurance relies on judgmental and subjective evaluations, whereas TQM emphasizes management by facts (numbers).

The quality scoring procedure involves an independent group of staff members assigned to coordinate and implement the quality assurance program. The following six specific objectives of the nursing process are taken into account.

1. Plan of care is formulated
2. Physical needs of the patients are met
3. Non-physical (psychosocial, emotional, and social) needs of the patients are met
4. Achievement of nursing care objectives is evaluated
5. Unit procedures are followed for the protection of all patients
6. Delivery of nursing care is facilitated by administrative and managerial services

Effective monitoring of patient care quality must begin with a complete understanding of who the customers are. This question is addressed next.

WHO IS THE CUSTOMER?

Hospitals, like many service organizations, have two categories of customers: external and internal. External customers include patients, physicians, families and friends, third party payers, and the community. Each customer group has a different list of criteria for evaluating the quality of care. Internal customers include departments and individuals that provide services to others (see Figure 3-1). A customer is not just the money-waving "ultimate" consumer of health-care resources. Anyone who you or your work unit provides service or information to is a customer.

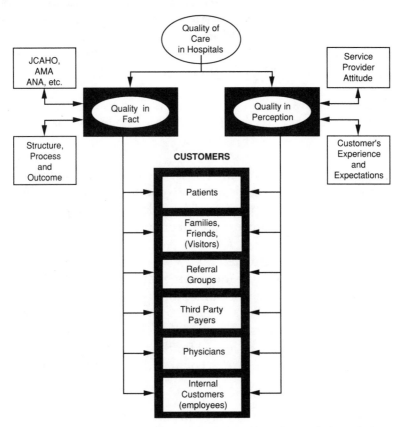

Figure 3-1. A conceptual framework for quality of care in hospitals.

After identifying the various customer groups in health-care organizations, it is essential to understand some of their quality requirements. Most of this section will be devoted to the patient, but first, we examine some of the quality requirements of the other class of customers. Physicians often evaluate quality in terms of many patient-related factors, such as promptness in receiving test results, timeliness of services to their patients, the degree of professionalism with which nurses carry out their orders, the completeness in the nurses' chart of patient status, and the presence of state-of-the-art technology.

The family members of patients may evaluate quality in terms of the factors that affect the patient as well as extraneous factors such as staff courtesy and degree of concern, cleanliness, and the flexibility of visitation policies. The payers on the other hand may be more concerned about accuracy of charges, promptness in billing, completeness of bill, etc. Since the patient is central to the activity of care delivery, the remaining material in this section will focus on the patient.

Quality of Care and the Patient

As a practical matter, a patient does not really care what the JCAHO manual says about quality, or whether or not an intravenous line is administered by a registered nurse or a licensed practical nurse. A patient perceives quality in the context of his or her own experience. It is not simply a question of whether health-care quality should be process or patient-oriented. Too often, the emphasis is placed on process quality, and as a result, the patient's perception of quality is overlooked.

According to King (1985), there are several theories that attempt to explain how customers evaluate the quality of service. The first theory states that there are two sides to the customer's perception of service quality. First, the primary or "core" service is performed, and second, that the surrounding or secondary services are performed satisfactorily. This theory holds that if the primary function is not performed satisfactorily, customer satisfaction cannot be recovered by high performance levels in the secondary functions.

The second theory separates the hard functions—the technology of the service—from the soft functions, the manner in which the service is performed. The customer's attitude toward a breakdown in the technology can be influenced by the manner in which such a situation is handled, but the effects of poor interactions with the service provider cannot be overcome by technically competent performance.

The third theory states that the service transaction is not a fixed entity, but rather a process, and the customer's evaluation of satisfaction can change over the course of the encounter.

A fourth theory pertains to the degree of perceived risk and the related cost of the service. The intangible nature of service presents a risk to the customer in that he cannot see and evaluate in advance what he is going to get. In addition, services performed generally involve either the customer personally or his property. When little risk or low cost is involved, customers apply less stringent standards of evaluation than when high risk or high cost is involved.

Each of these four theories will now be examined in the context of quality in health care. For example, from the first theory, the two sides of a patient's perception of quality may be stated as follows:

- *Primary service:* Was the surgery performed correctly or successfully?

- *Secondary service:* Were the nurses friendly? Was the billing accurate? Were the bed linens changed regularly?

Very often, hospital, clinical, and administrative staff will define quality in the context of the primary service alone. However, the fact remains that patients generally expect a hospital to have competent and professionally trained clinicians who will follow the proper procedures in their work. Except for patients who are familiar with the workings of a hospital, most patients do not know what constitutes a "proper procedure." What patients do know and can respond to is the manner in which a service is performed (for example, the behavior of the individuals providing the service). The quality of the interaction between the care provider and recipient is critical in health care. King calls this factor the "quality of behavior." According to Johnson (1988),

> Despite all the new technology in hospitals, health care remains a humanistic activity. People's experiences at the hands of a health-care professional in times of vulnerability are intensely personal. A patient needs that

human touch, caring, and compassion. Consumers have come to expect not only the latest technology and highly competent professionals, but a care-giving culture as well.

In many cases, patients change physicians, nurses, clinics, and even hospitals, not because of the poor clinical quality but because of poor "quality of behavior." Health care is a humanistic profession and the labor involved is a labor of love. Hochschild (1983) refers to this type of labor as "emotional labor" to distinguish it from physical labor and mental labor. Health-care dollars do not only buy the medical expertise and ability of the practitioners, but also their attitude.

The second theory concludes that technical or clinical expertise cannot compensate for a care giver's poor interaction with the patient or other non-care activity. However, good quality interactions with the recipient of service may positively influence a patient when there is inadequacy in the technical aspects. A quality program must give sufficient attention to the hard (technical) functions as well as the soft (non-technical) functions of the care delivery process. Quality should not be judged only in terms of the visible aspects of patient services. Many of the services provided to the patient are not seen. Examples of such "invisible" services are medical records and information management. Still, there are other services which the patient cannot evaluate while care is being provided, but will have the opportunity of evaluating later, e.g. billing and follow-up care. Quality must be viewed in the context of a patient's total experience.

The premise of the third theory is somewhat similar to what Albrecht and Zemke describe as "moment of truth" in their book *Service America* (1985). The term "moment of truth," originally coined by Jan Carlzon, president of Scandinavian Airlines, is defined as "any episode in which the customer comes into contact with any aspect of the organization and gets an impression of the quality of its service."

According to this definition, every "moment of truth" provides an opportunity for the care provider to make a good impression on the care recipient, and thus influence the evaluation of care received by the patient. The implication is that if you as a provider of service get it wrong at your point in a patient's chain of experiences, you will likely erase from the patient's mind any other good experiences he or she may have had before the encounter with you. But if you get it right, you have a chance to undo all the wrong things that may have occurred during the patient's experience prior to you. You really are the "moment of truth" in the Provider-Receiver (PR) encounter. When PR encounters go unmanaged, the quality of service deteriorates to unacceptable levels.

This point can be further illustrated by examining a hospital whose emergency room is divided into six departments as follows:

1. The initial examination station to treat minor problems or make diagnosis (INITIAL EXAM)
2. An X-ray department (X-RAY)
3. An operating room
4. A cast fitting room
5. An observation room for recovery and general observation before the final diagnosis or release
6. An out-processing department where clerks check patients out and arrange for payment or insurance forms

A patient in this example can be expected to have anywhere from two to four PR encounters during a visit to the emergency room. The patient's perception can be altered or influenced by any contact made in any of the six departments of the emergency room.

Failure to adequately manage PR encounters may often lead to patient abuse and neglect particularly in nursing homes. Rosander (1985) notes that patient abuse and neglect (in nursing home care) include a wide variety of practices: removing trays before meals are eaten, threatening slow eaters, delays in answering the call light, refusing to give patients something they like to eat such as a slice of bread, isolating patients in a corridor and leaving them for hours, refusing to talk to patients, or employees taking long coffee breaks regardless of the patients' needs. An understanding of the expectations of the customers is a necessary starting point in defining the needs of customers.

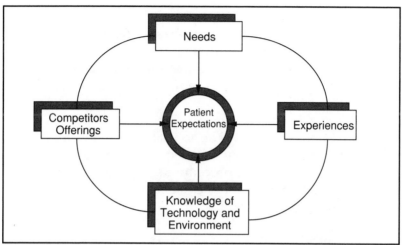

Figure 3-2. Factors affecting patient expectations.

Patient Expectations

The expectations of patients are influenced by the following components as depicted in Figure 3-2.

- *Needs:* The need to alleviate a health-related problem, be cured, or slow the growth process of a certain illness, is critical in the definition of patient expectations.

- *Experiences:* What the customer has encountered (in the past) in the delivery of health care.

- *Knowledge of technology and environment:* How much the patient knows about what types of services are available, the scope of such services including risks, and the technological level at which the services are available. Also important is knowledge of the experiences of others such as relatives, friends, and visitors.

- *Competitors' offerings:* The knowledge of what other health-care organizations are offering, or promising to offer, can have a tremendous impact on the expectations of customers.

In order to fully understand patient expectations, it is help-ful to categorize them in three phases: before going to the hospital, during hospital visit, and after leaving the hospital. The following are examples of the expectations of a person going into the hospital for a procedure:

Before entering hospital:
• The condition/disease will be accurately diagnosed
• The condition/disease will be adequately explained
• The risks inherent in the procedure(s) will be explained
• Charges will be satisfactorily explained
• The information given will be reliable and complete

During hospital stay:
• The procedure will be performed by a team of competent medical and nursing professionals
• The procedure will take place as promised, predicted, or explained
• The medical and nursing staff will show compassion, warmth, and care during hospitalization
• The recovery will progress as predicted, promised, or ex-plained
• The staff will do everything possible to bring about complete recovery
• An acceptable level of hygiene and cleanliness will be ob-served by the hospital staff
• Meals will be served at an acceptable temperature, in ad-equate quantity, with proper nutritional balance, and at the right time
• Call lights will be answered promptly
• He/she will get better or be cured
• Instructions for rehabilitation and medication will be clear and complete

After leaving the hospital:
• There will not be a repeat visit to the hospital for the same problem
• The bill from the hospital and professional staff will be accu-rate and adequately explained
• Recovery will take place as explained

- The hospital and its professional staff will respond promptly if problems develop again

Consumer Behavior

Peters and Waterman (1984) emphasize the importance of "staying close to the customer." By this they mean a deliberate probe into what quality requirements are important to customers. What will they spend money on? What will they not spend money on? In a study of consumer behavior carried out by Technical Assistance Research Programs, Inc. (TARP) for the White House Office of Consumer Affairs, the following are some of the published findings:

- The average business never hears from 96 percent of its unhappy customers. For every complaint received, the average company has approximately 26 customers with problems.

- Complainers are more likely than noncomplainers to do business again with the company that upset them, even if the problem is not satisfactorily resolved.

- Of the customers that make a complaint, between 54 and 70 percent will do business again with the organization when the matter is resolved. If the matter is resolved quickly, the figure goes up to 95 percent.

- The average customer who has had a problem with an organization will tell nine to ten people about it.

- Customers who have complained to an organization and had their complaints satisfactorily resolved tell an average of five people about the treatment they received.

Several studies have suggested that an increasing number of health-care consumers are obtaining their information from friends and relatives (see Table 3-1).

Although the influence of physicians over patients remains strong in the selection of hospitals, more patients are insisting on having a say in matters affecting hospital selection. Figure 3-

Table 3-1. Sources of health-care information. *(Reprinted from Hospitals, Vol. 63, No. 16, by permission, August 20, 1989, Copyright 1989, American Hospital Publishing, Inc.)*

Sources of health-care information	1984	1985	1986	1987/88	1989
Friend/relative	27.0%	25.6%	17.8%	28.1%	49.9%
Family physician	45.8%	41.1%	50.4%	43.8%	20.8%
Newspaper	10.9%	11.4%	7.6%	5.4%	4.6%
Hospital mailings	3.1%	3.0%	4.0%	3.8%	3.7%
Work	0.0%	3.7%	3.5%	0.0%	2.8%
Other	13.2%	15.2%	16.7%	18.9%	18.2%

3 shows the results of a survey on how patients might respond to the recommendations of their physicians towards the selection of hospitals.

As Figure 3-3 indicates, although the influence of the physician remains very strong, a growing number of the patients surveyed are likely to change physicians if the wrong hospital is recommended for them. Parkland Associates conducted a study of patient data from nearly 200 hospitals in 43 states which revealed that nursing care is the most important factor patients consider when recommending a hospital (*AHA News* 1990).

Leebov (1988) identifies four primary reasons why health-care organizations should focus on a patient's perception and satisfaction with the services provided:

- *The humanistic reason:* Patients deserve excellent quality of care and service because they are often quite vulnerable. They come with anxiety about their physical, emotional, and economic well-being. Excellent service not only enhances quality of care, but also helps allay the anxiety that comes with being hospitalized.

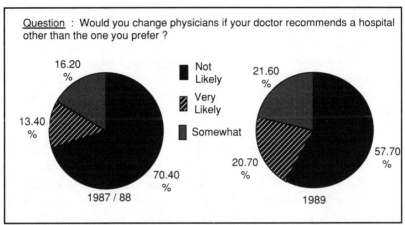

Question : Would you change physicians if your doctor recommends a hospital other than the one you prefer ?

■ Not Likely

▨ Very Likely

▮ Somewhat

1987 / 88

1989

Figure 3-3. Physician's recommmendations and reactions. *(Reprinted from Hospitals, Vol. 63, No. 16, by permission, August 20, 1989, American Hospital Publishing, Inc.)*

• *The economic reason:* Patients are customers. They now have more options and are expecting value for their money.

• *The marketing reason:* Patients can be good or bad for public relations depending upon the experiences they have while receiving services.

• *The efficiency reason:* Satisfied patients are easier to serve, whereas dissatisfied patients consume more valuable staff time that could be used serving others.

THE QUALITY OF BEHAVIOR

In a 1985 Gallup survey for the American Society for Quality Control, it was revealed that employee behavior and attitudes are the major determinant of the quality of services. The survey was based on interviews with 1,005 persons. Rosander (1989) identified three classes of human traits that can affect quality of service. They are behavior, attitudes, and appearance. Using the examples suggested by Rosander, the following cases are developed for health care on two of these three classes.

Behavior

- *Acting promptly:* A patient (or patient's family member) should be able to see promptness in response to pain, to a request, to a patient's call for assistance, or to a need. This attribute is critical for nurses, physicians, laboratory testing services, the pharmacy, etc.

- *Listening carefully:* Sometimes physicians are perceived as not listening enough to their patients. A patient or family member should be able to perceive the doctor as one who listens attentively to health-related complaints and questions. It is equally important for nurses to be careful listeners to the patients and also for nurses and physicians to listen carefully to each other, especially in matters affecting the patient.

- *Being attentive:* For a patient whose life is on the line, being attentive is not just an indication of good quality, it is a critical attribute. The need to be attentive is especially critical during the performance of surgical operations, administering medication (oral or intravenously), and monitoring cardiac activity.

- *Acting with understanding:* Nursing is a humanistic profession—one that calls for understanding and compassion on the part of the provider of care. The provider of care must act in a manner that shows empathy with the pain and suffering of the afflicted. When a nurse says to a screaming patient, "You don't have to scream at me; I didn't cause your injury," it defies understanding and compassion.

- *Making "to-the-point" explanations:* Nurses are expected to demonstrate sufficient knowledge of their jobs in a manner that allows them to provide precise and adequate explanation to patients, relatives, and physicians. It is not always easy to provide a to-the-point explanation to the family of a patient whose chance of survival after an operation is less than desirable.

- *Avoiding unusual ways of talking:* Appropriate linguistic skills on the part of the service provider is often perceived as good quality by the customer. This is no less true in health care. Nurses, physicians, nursing unit support services staff, and X-ray and laboratory technicians are all expected to avoid unusual ways of talking around or away from the patients and their relatives.

- *Showing ability to do the job:* When a service provider demonstrates a lack of confidence and knowledge, he or she is usually perceived as not possessing the ability to do the job. Sometimes after consecutive 12-hour shifts, fatigue sets in and it becomes harder to demonstrate "ability."

- *Getting along with people:* In general, customers perceive the ability to get along with people (on the part of the provider of service) as an indication of the presence of quality in the service being delivered.

Attitudes

The components of attitudes include being courteous, friendly, mannerly, kind, conversational, alert, accurate, responsible, and compassionate.

Appearance

Appearance denotes a visual impression of the way a person or thing is or seems. Although appearance focuses on the outward aspects of a person or thing, it is often true that customer perception may be affected by such factors. The appearance of the nursing staff, the inpatient and outpatient facilities, the reception area, etc., are all very important elements of perceived quality.

Reports from Health-Care Surveys

An article by Mary Koska in *Hospitals* (1989), reports the results of a survey of 663 hospital chief executive officers (CEOs). The survey was conducted by the consulting firm of Hamilton/KSA from Atlanta, Georgia. The survey asked CEOs to rank, in order of significance, ten factors that contribute to a hospital's quality of care. The results of this survey are presented in Table 3-2 .

Table 3-2. CEO survey: What are the most significant factors in providing high quality care? (Ranked by how frequently a factor was mentioned as one of the top three contributors to quality.) *(Reprinted from Hospitals, Vol. 63, No. 3, by permission, February 5, 1989. Copyright 1989, American Hospital Publishing, Inc.)*

97.3%	Nursing care
96.4%	Clinical skills of medical staff
93.3%	Employee attitudes
89.9%	State-of-the-art technology
85.6%	Hospital administration
82.1%	Internal operations
74.9%	Appearance of physical facility
69.0%	Convenience/access
61.0%	Food service
52.8%	Board involvement in quality assurance

Koska reported Barry Moore, president of Hamilton/KSA, as saying, "Truly effective nursing care has two parts—the clinical component and the caring component—neither of which can stand alone and still be considered high-quality care." According to Moore, "It's almost impossible for patients to measure technical quality. They generally assume it will be there...on the other hand, what patients can easily measure, they can criticize." For example, food service, which was ranked as a significant contributor to high-quality care by 61 percent of CEOs surveyed, may be the quickest way to impress patients. According to Moore, poor food service, noise, inadequate explanations, and rudeness of the staff are the most common complaints that patients have about hospitals.

Steiber of SRI Gallup Poll (1988) reports the results of a national poll conducted for *Hospitals* magazine, in which consumer satisfaction was found to be influenced more by concern shown for the patient than by clinical care. The 414 respondents had either been hospitalized themselves within the past two years or had immediate family members who had been hospitalized. According to Steiber, traditional analyses of patient satisfaction generally look only at how patients rate different services, such as food, cleanliness and parking. But these scores only tell hospital executives how well the hospital performs those individual tasks. Such surveys do not indicate the degree to which consumers associate these services with quality of care. Steiber notes that, "The single most important action hospital executives can take to maintain quality from the patient's perspective is to deliver a satisfactory experience."

It should be pointed out that hospitals should expect patients to use stringent standards of evaluation regardless of whether the risks and costs are high. King's (1985) fourth theory would therefore seem inappropriate because, even if a given patient's risk or cost is low, the patient's willingness to return for service or to refer another person to the hospital remains in jeopardy. Any attempt to emphasize only one aspect of quality (conformance or perception) at the expense of the other will be a disservice to the patient. What is needed is a total service quality management perspective.

MOVING TOWARD A TOTAL SERVICE QUALITY MANAGEMENT PROCESS

According to Albrecht and Zemke (1988), service management is a total organizational approach that makes quality of service, as perceived by the customer, the number one driving force for the operation of the business. If hospitals are to become competitive and guarantee themselves long-term survival, they should look more closely at the concept of Total Service Quality Management (TSQM). The following definition of TSQM is offered:

TSQM is a concept that defines quality in the context of a customer's experience. The customer's experience and subsequent perception of quality is affected by both the tangible and the intangible components of the services provided as well as what happens after the customer departs physically from the system providing the service. TSQM begins with top management commitment and must be instituted at all levels of the organization.

Critical Factors in TSQM

Total Service Quality Management is not a departmental activity. It is a hospital-wide concept embedded in every aspect of patient care. It is not an exclusive function of the "customer service department" nor the "patient complaints department." Everyone has a responsibility to ensure that things turn out right for the patient or the customer. Unfortunately, as most QA departments in hospitals learn, the implication of departmentalizing QA is that some employees feel that they can afford to mess up since there is a central department that can fix their mistakes. Notwithstanding, the whole organization should act like one huge customer service or quality assurance department.

A hospital is typically managed on the basis of individual functions such as nursing, pharmacy, and housekeeping. Consequently, no single individual or group is really accountable for building quality into the patient's experience. This is perhaps the most compelling reason why the TSQM concept should encompass every individual and every level in the organization.

Successful hospitals and health-care organizations begin with quality, not cost, in evaluating the effectiveness of their care delivery operation. When quality is high, demand goes up, costs go down, and productivity and profits go up (refer to Figure 3-4). The end result is higher profits and satisfied customers. Unsuccessful health-care organizations, on the other hand, tend to be fearfully and nervously preoccupied with cost reduction and profit-maximization, hoping that quality will just happen. With more and more hospitals employing administrators who have business and finance degrees, the idea of ignor-

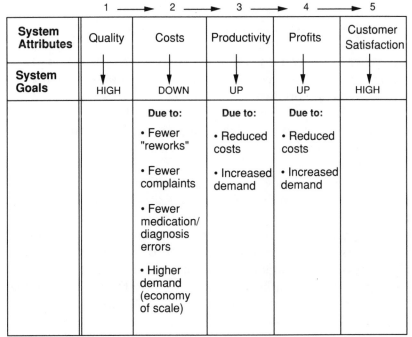

Figure 3-4. System attributes and relationships.

ing costs and focusing on quality seems preposterous. It is a very difficult concept to grasp. An increase in quality yields a decrease in costs only if quality refers to uniformity. But an increase in quality yields an increase in costs if quality refers to features.

Service is not only a potent weapon in a hospital's competitive arsenal; it is the driving force behind profitability. Productivity must be seen as a subset of quality. What is needed now is a new paradigm—one that reverses the old emphasis on cost reduction and productivity. Hospitals can only become or remain profitable if they first identify the right things and then do them right. Johnson (1988) notes that, "Hospitals are much more than buildings and machines, they are human organizations meeting human needs; and to remain successful in a competitive health-care market, they must outperform their competitors on the human dimension."

Knowing your customers and how they rate you is another critical factor in TSQM. Market research has proved to be a powerful tool in gathering information about the patient. It is critical to know what the patients who use your hospital think of your service. It is equally important to know who the patients are, where they come from, and why they come to you. This information can help you to determine how much of the hospital market your organization controls and how your hospital ranks among the other competing hospitals. The market research must seek to establish which factors people really consider most important during their visits to or stays in your hospital.

Also of importance is knowing how your hospital compares to other hospitals on these factors. It is dangerous to rely solely on hospital management's opinions of patient perceptions. Hospital administrators may fail to recognize that the patient's needs have evolved in response either to the competitive standards of other hospitals or to environmental influences. Once this information is gathered, a hospital must then chart a course to meet and surpass the expectations of its customers.

Marketing Research

Once a health-care organization has answered the questions from the preceding section—who are its customers and what are their wants and needs—it must determine how it is rated against its competitors, and, if necessary, what it must do to win over the customer. There is only one way to convince the customer that your organization is better; it is by offering a service that meets or surpasses the expectation of the customer and providing a service that is decisively superior to what the competitors are offering. It is important to determine for example, why some physicians do not recommend your hospital to their patients, or why certain patient groups perceive your nurses as being unfriendly (when compared to the other hospitals), or how your emergency room services compare against that of your competitors (in the eyes of the customers).

Marketing research involves the systematic gathering, recording, and analyzing of information about specific issues affecting the product or services being provided. It is the information link between the customer and the provider of the service. Marketing research should be based on objectivity, accuracy, and completeness. Objectivity means that the research is conducted in an unbiased and open-minded manner. Accuracy refers to the use of valid research tools and/or instruments that are carefully constructed. Each aspect of research, such as the sample chosen, questionnaire format, and tabulation of responses, must be carefully planned. Completeness refers to the comprehensive nature of the research. Erroneous conclusions may be reached if the research does not probe deeply or widely enough.

When, for example, a hospital asks its patients to rate its (the hospital's) parking facility on a scale of 1 to 5 (1 being poor, and 5 being excellent), what exactly is it asking? It is merely asking its patients to rate how well it is doing with respect to parking, but not necessarily asking whether or not parking is important to the patient, or for that matter how important parking is compared to, for example, warm meals. It is advisable to hire the services of an outside research firm if a health-care organization finds that it does not have the in-house capability to carry out good market research.

A radial diagram is a useful tool for depicting how a hospital stacks up against its competition. To prepare a radial diagram, a hospital selects the quality characteristics by which it is judged against its competitors. The hospital's customers (patients, doctors, etc.) provide a rating from 1 to 5 (5 being the highest) for the various quality characteristics. A radial diagram, such as that in Figure 3-5, provides a visual representation of how your hospital has performed against the competition, and also depicts areas in need of improvement.

Other Customers

Besides patients, hospitals have other customers, both internal and external that are often ignored. External customers include families and friends of patients, insurance companies and other payers, physicians, and other outside health-care agencies.

Internal customers include the staff from various departments who rely on output from one another in order to complete their work. For example, a physician relies on output from the laboratory department before making a diagnosis. The goal

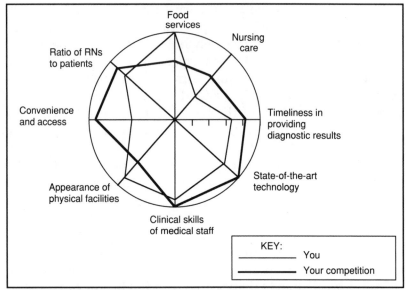

Figure 3-5. Radial diagram showing how you stand against your competition.

must be to understand and strive to meet the needs of both internal and external customers.

The concept of TSQM in health care can be grasped more easily if adequate attempts are first made to understand some of its theoretical foundations. The theoretical foundations are presented below in what is referred to as the Twelve Quality Dimensions of Today's Health-Care Business.

THE TWELVE QUALITY DIMENSIONS OF TODAY'S HEALTH-CARE BUSINESS

1. Whether the DRG program continues or not, the issues of quality, productivity, technology, and competitiveness will continue to be important in the health-care business.

2. Today's health-care customers, including patients, relatives, and doctors, are thought to be more sensitive to quality differences and their choice of facilities will be affected accordingly.

3. High (perceived or technical) quality is expected to produce greater customer loyalty. Over time, that should translate into an increased rate of return visits and referrals to health-care organizations.

4. An undisputable connection between quality and productivity exists.

5. Quality is not a departmental activity; it is everybody's responsibility, including nurses, doctors, nursing unit support services, pharmacy, and biomedical technicians.

6. Patient (customer) satisfaction is affected by competitive offerings and should be evaluated at the time of the hospital visit and again following discharge.

7. Conformance to standards (JCAHO) appears to become a secondary concern, to be pursued only after the needs of the hospital's customers have been carefully defined.

8. If quality and profitability are so closely linked, hospitals must strive to meet and exceed the level of quality demonstrated by their competitors.

9. It is not enough to be doing all the right things well, hospitals also have to do them better with respect to the competition.

10. The services provided by other hospitals (competitors) should be studied to establish what customers mean when they say one hospital, facility, or service is of higher quality than another.

11. Competitors are not likely to sit back and watch their superiority being challenged or surpassed; they too will strive to improve quality. Quality will then become an upward moving target, which will reset continually at higher and higher levels.

12. Continuous improvement should become the deliberate objective rather than the achievement of an acceptable quality level based on internal standards or JCAHO requirements.

A hospital is a service organization; therefore, it performs rather than produces. To survive and prosper in the health-care industry requires differentiation. A hospital must show evidence that it really does have something special to offer.

Quality assurance is not a departmental activity. The responsibility for quality lies with everyone—from the secretary who avoids typing errors, to the hospital's telephone operator who must effectively handle the inquiries of potential patients and their relatives and friends, to the nurse who must enter correct and accurate information into patient charts and avoid medication errors, and so on. No hospital can evade this quality challenge: profit-making or non-profit hospitals, general or specialist hospitals, private or public hospitals, government or nongovernment. All must face the task of responding effectively and efficiently to patients who expect quality service in the delivery of care as part of the hospital's product. Some hospitals are well-aware of this need and are generating measured responses. For many others, the need to be patient-centered and service-quality driven comes as a major surprise. Nevertheless, this need cannot be ignored; it is not a whimsical trend that will suddenly disappear. It is the new standard by which today's patients measure the performance of health-care organizations.

It may be useful to envision the patient as carrying around a mental "report card," in which he or she records a perceived score for the services received from the system. This score helps the patient decide whether to come back for this service or go to another hospital, and whether or not to recommend a particular hospital to someone else. As hospitals move into a new era of competitiveness, it is critical that they learn as much as possible about the all-important, but invisible, report card. In the final analysis, a hospital's ability to consistently score impressive marks on the patient's report card ultimately depends on how much the hospital knows about the patient's evaluation criteria.

It is not those who provide the service, but those whom it serves, who have the final word on how well the service fulfills needs and expectations.

EXERCISES

3-1. Give a list of five customer quality requirements that can be categorized as soft and hard factors.

3-2. What mechanisms are in place at your facility for obtaining feedback from your health-care customers?

3-3. How does your organization determine the requirements of its internal customers?

3-4. When was the last time your organization conducted a survey to determine how it performs against its competition?

BIBLIOGRAPHY

Accreditation Manual for Hospitals. 1990. Chicago, IL: Joint Commission on Accreditation of Hospital Organizations. p. 310.

AHA News. 1990. Chicago, IL: American Hospital Association, 26(49).

Albrecht, K. and R. Zemke. 1985. *Service America.* Homewood, IL: Dow Jones Irwin Publishers.

American Nurses' Association. 1973. *Standards for Nursing Services.* Kansas City, MO: American Nurses ' Association.

Aydelotte, M. K. 1973. Staffing for high quality care. *Hospitals.* (January 16) 43:58-60.

Batchelor, G. J. and R. Graham. 1989. Quality management in nursing. *Journal of the Society for Health Systems.* 1(1):63.

Bennett, A. C. 1983. *Productivity and the Quality of Work Life in Hospitals.* Chicago, IL: American Hospital Association.

Crosby, P. B. 1979. *Quality is Free.* New York: Mc-Graw Hill Book Co.

Day, R. G. 1988. Quality cost and productivity. *Quality Progress.* (July) p. 59.

Donabedian, A. 1976. Some basic issues in evaluating the quality of care. *Issues in Evaluation Research.* New York: American Nurses' Association. Pub. no. G1224M. p. 7.

_____. 1980. *The Definition of Quality and Approaches to Its Assessment. Vol. 1. Explorations in Quality Assurance and Monitoring.* Ann Arbor, MI: Health Administration Press.

Egdahl, R. and P. Gertman. 1976. *Quality Assurance in Health Care.* Rockville, MD: Aspen Publishers.

Franz, J. 1984. Challenge for nursing: Hiking productivity without lowering quality of care. *Modern Healthcare.* (September) pp. 60-68.

Garvin, D. A. 1988. *Managing Quality.* New York: The Free Press.

Graham, N. 1982. *Quality Assurance in Hospitals: Strategies for Assessment and Implementation.* Rockville, MD: Aspen Publishers.

Hostage, G. M. 1975. Quality control in a service business. *Harvard Business Review.* (July-August).

Hochschild, A. R. 1983. *The Managed Heart: The Commercialization of Human Feeling.* Berkeley, CA: University of California Press.

Jelinek, R. C., R. Dieter Haussman, S. Hegyvary, and J. Newman, Jr. 1974. *A Methodology for Monitoring Quality of Nursing Care.*

Washington, DC: Government Printing Office. DHEW Pub. no. (HRA) 76-25.

Johnson, J. A. 1988. Service management, a strategy for excellence in health care. *Business Perspectives.* (July) p. 13.

King, C. A. 1985. Service quality assurance is different. *Quality Progress,* 18(6):14.

Koska, M. T. 1989. Quality—thy name is nursing care, CEOs say. *Hospitals.* 63(3):32.

Leebov, W. 1988. *Service Excellence: The Customer Relations Strategy for Health Care.* Chicago, IL: American Hospital Publishing, Inc.

Luke, R. D., J. Krueger, and R. Modrow. 1983. *Organization and Change in Health Care Quality Assurance.* Rockville, MD: Aspen Publications.

Meisenheimer, C. G., ed. 1985. *Quality Assurance : A Complete Guide to Effective Programs.* Rockville, MD: Aspen Publications.

Millenson, M. L. 1987. A prescription for change. *Quality Progress.* 5:18.

Miller, M. C. and R. Knapp. 1979. *Evaluating Quality of Care.* Gaithersburg, MD: Aspen Systems Corp.

Miller, M. C. and R. Knapp. 1979. *Evaluating Quality of Care: Analytical Procedures, Monitoring Techniques.* Germantown, MD: Aspen Publishers.

Mowry, M. M. and R. Korpman. 1986. *Managing Health Care Costs, Quality, and Technology: Product Line Strategies for Nursing.* Rockville, MD: Aspen Publishers.

Omachonu, V. K. 1990. Quality of care and the patient: New criteria for evaluation. *Health Care Management Review.* 15:4.

Omachonu, V. K. and R. Nanda. 1988. IEs in health care management must emphasize client-centered projects which can contain cost while supporting quality. *Industrial Engineering.* Norcross, GA: Institute of Industrial Engineers. 20:10.

Omachonu, V. K. and M. Beruvides. 1989. Improving hospital productivity: Patient-, unit-, and hospital-based measures. *International Industrial Engineering Conference Proceedings.* Norcross, GA: Institute of Industrial Engineers.

Peters, T. J. and R. H. Waterman, Jr. 1984. *In Search of Excellence.* New York: Warner Books.

Rosander, A. C. 1989. *The Quest for Quality in Services.* Milwaukee, WI: Quality Press and White Plains, NY: Quality Resources. p. 55.

Rosander, A. C. 1988. *Applications of Quality Control in the Service Industries.* Milwaukee, WI: Quality Press and White Plains, NY: Marcel Dekker, Inc.

Rush-Presbyterian-St. Luke's Medical Center and Medicus Systems Corporation. 1974. *A Methodology for Evaluation of Quality of Life and Care in Long-Term Care Facilities.* Chicago, IL: Medicus.

Sahney, V. K., J. Dutkewych and W. Schramm. 1989. Quality improvement process: The foundation for excellence in health care. *Journal of the Society for Health Systems.* 1(1):17.

Sasser, W. E., R. Olsen and D. Wyckoff. 1978. *Management of Service Operations, Text and Cases.* Allyn and Bacon, Inc. p. 180.

Schroeder, P. and M. Regina. 1984. *Nursing Quality Assurance: A Unit-Based Approach.* Gaithersburg, MD: Aspen Systems Corp.

Steiber, S. R. 1988. How consumers perceive health care quality. *Hospitals.* (April 5) p. 84.

Thompson, P., G. DeSouza, and B. Gale. 1985. Strategic management of service quality. *Quality Progress.* (June) p. 20.

Townsend, P. L. 1985. Insurance firm shows that quality has value. *Quality Progress.* (June) p. 42.

Ullmann, S. G. 1985. The impact of quality on cost in the provision of long-term care. *Inquiry.* 22:293-302.

U.S. Office of Consumer's Affairs. 1986. Complaint handling in America. TARP, Inc.

Werner, J. P. 1988. Measuring quality in the health care delivery business: Can it be done? *Industrial Management.* Norcross, GA: Institute of Industrial Engineers. 30(5):22.

4 Total Service Quality Management

Today, more than any other time in our history, health-care organizations are showing concern over issues such as quality, cost, and competitiveness.

The imperatives of competition dictate that a hospital whose current status is poor must improve rapidly if it is to survive. One whose status is superior must improve to preserve its competitive edge, and a hospital which is average must improve to prevent its status from regressing to poor and to make it superior. The current status of a hospital organization can always be improved. The relationships linking Total Service Quality Management (TSQM), productivity, and technology will become evident as the present theories and tools of TSQM are presented in this chapter.

THEORIES ABOUT QUALITY

Quality According to Crosby

Phillip B. Crosby gained a great deal of attention after the release of his book *Quality Is Free* (1979). At the time of the book's release, he was a corporate vice president and the director of quality at ITT. Currently, he is a quality management consultant.

Crosby points out that organizations bear an enormous cost burden by not doing the job right the first time. He describes the hidden costs of poor quality as consisting of increased labor and machine hours, increased machine failures and downtime, customer delivery delays and lost future sales, and increased warranty costs. These cost components are over and above the loss of materials to scrap. He actively advocates a goal of zero defects and subscribes to the use of continuous improvement as a means of achieving zero defects. Crosby notes that building quality into a product does not cost the company more. In fact, savings in rework, scrap, and servicing the product after the sale are benefits of quality design. In addition, there are the benefits of customer satisfaction and repeat sales.

Crosby defines quality as conformance to requirements. He stresses the following ideas :

- The system should emphasize prevention rather than checking and inspection. Inspection is wasteful.

- Prevention involves identifying areas where errors can occur, and once identified, the process should be modified to permanently eliminate the causes.

- The ultimate goal in quality management is to reach "zero defects."

- The cost of quality is the cost of doing things wrong.

- The price of non-conformance can be as high as 25-35 percent of organization operating costs.

- Prevention costs include the cost of quality-related education, training, preventive maintenance, process change, and process design.

In his book *Quality Without Tears* (1984), Crosby gives the following 14 steps in a quality improvement program.

1. Management's commitment
2. Quality improvement team
3. Quality measurement
4. The cost of quality
5. Quality awareness
6. Corrective action
7. Zero defects planning
8. Employee education and training
9. Zero defects day
10. Goal settings
11. Error-cause removal
12. Recognition
13. Quality councils
14. Doing it all over again

Quality According to Deming

Dr. W. Edwards Deming, author of *Out of the Crises* (1986), is the American statistician credited with the revitalization of the Japanese economy in the 1950s. There are many who give Deming the credit for bringing the war-ravaged Japan to its current respectable and dominant status in world trade. In 1951, the Japanese Union of Scientists and Engineers (JUSE) established the Deming Prizes, in honor of Dr. Deming for his contributions in the area of quality control. The prizes are awarded annually. The research and education prize goes to individuals, and the prize for applications goes to corporations or plants that have demonstrated outstanding results in the improvement of quality. In 1989, Florida Power and Light Company became the first non-Japanese company to win the Deming prize.

Considered to be the father of quality control in Japan, Dr. Deming, like Crosby, asserts that achieving excellence in quality starts with top management. Deming notes that management must develop the proper theory and tools to manage quality. He believes that building quality into a product leads to lower costs and hence improvement in productivity and competitive position. Dr. Deming describes two types of variations in a process—special and system variation. Special variations are caused by meaningful factors to be investigated. They are avoidable and cannot be ignored. System (also referred to as common) variations are variations due to chance; they are unavoidable and inevitably occur in a process. Common variations include mistakes, complaints, accidents, etc.

Dr. Deming condemns the idea of speaking of quality as though it means "doing one's best." Everyone doing his best is not the answer. People must first understand the nature of the transformation necessary in American organizations. Deming remarks that employees should not be held accountable for job behavior or for the results expected of them. Deming condemns the concepts of performance appraisal, management by objectives, management by numbers, and work standards. He feels such concepts are destructive, inhibit self actualization, and destroy pride in workmanship. Dr. Deming deplores the notion of "more of the same," adding that there is no substitute for knowledge. Management must not be misled into thinking that a figure or number constitutes knowledge. It is possible to meet specifications and yet not improve the satisfaction level of the product or service. Recognition of the difference between a stable system and an unstable one is important in the effective management of an organization. A stable system is one whose performance is predictable or in statistical control. Only management can reduce the problems that exist in a stable system. Deming calls for the continuous improvement of design and processes at the source.

Deming believes that management has failed in the United States. He makes the following observations (Mann 1989):

> The emphasis is on the quick buck, while the emphasis in Japan is to plan decades ahead. The next quarterly dividend is not as important as existence of the company 5, 10, or 20 years from now. One requirement for innovation is faith that there will be a future.

Deming proposed a 14-point plan, which will help top-level management to improve productivity, competitive position, and stay in business. Deming's plan stresses the following ideas:

• Quality must be built into the process.

• Statistical methods should be used rather than 100 percent inspection. Mass inspection implies that a process cannot produce defect-free items.

Excerpted from *Out of Crises*, Deming's 14 points are listed below.

1. Create constancy of purpose for improvement of product and service.
2. Adopt the new philosophy.
3. Cease dependence on inspection to achieve quality.
4. End the practice of awarding business on the basis of price tag alone. Instead, minimize total cost by working with a single supplier.
5. Improve constantly and forever every process for planning, production, and service.
6. Institute training on the job.
7. Adopt and institute leadership.
8. Drive out fear.
9. Break down barriers between staff areas.
10. Eliminate slogans, exhortations, and targets for the work force.
11. Eliminate numerical quotas for the work force and numerical goals for management.
12. Remove barriers that rob people of pride of workmanship. Eliminate the annual rating or merit system.
13. Institute a vigorous program of education and self-improvement for everyone.
14. Put everybody in the company to work to accomplish the transformation.

Deming's 14 Points Applied To Health-Care Organizations

Point 1: Create constancy of purpose. Hospitals need to create constancy of purpose in the quest for continuous improvement of technical quality and the customer perception of quality. The hospital's organizational philosophy should reflect this total commitment to constantly improving quality in all ways. Constancy of purpose requires that hospitals embrace the opportunities of tomorrow by charting the course today. Without a clear vision of the future, it is doubtful that a health-care organization will achieve its goal. As surprising as it may seem, there are many hospitals that do not have a mission statement. While a mission statement is not an end in itself, it can be a perpetual reminder of *constancy of purpose.*

Point 2: *Adopt the new philosophy for a changing economic age.* The top-level management of hospitals will have to launch their organizations into a new economic age; one that recognizes the need to meet and surpass the expectations of customers. Some of the elements of the new age are as follows:

• The "customers" of a hospital are not just patients, but also physicians, third party payers, patients' relatives and friends, etc.

• Each customer group possesses a list of quality requirements that cannot be ignored.

• The expectations of today's health-care "customers" are higher and greatly affect the satisfaction level for services received.

• The challenge facing health-care administrators today is how to achieve an optimum balance between high quality care and cost containment.

• Organizational policies should be driven by a clear understanding of the needs of today's health-care customers and the present environment. Quality does not only mean compliance to JCAHO's requirements; it means learning and applying many concepts, ideas, and tools in a process of continuous improvement.

• Cooperation is better than competition. Competition leads to a win-lose situation while cooperation leads to a win-win situation. By cooperating, everybody wins, and so does society as a whole.

Point 3: *Cease dependence on mass inspection.* Mass inspection cannot undo the damage caused by administering the wrong medication or a patient becoming infected during hospitalization. Emphasis should be on process improvement and the elimination of problems that compromise quality of care. Because hospital organizations purchase a variety of items such as drugs, food, and ancillary supplies, sometimes inspection is necessary. Hospitals need to work together with reputable vendors and suppliers to ensure compliance to acceptable quality levels.

Point 4: *Cease buying based on price tag alone.* The need to cease buying based on the price tag alone is especially important in health care, where drugs, instruments, equipment, and supplies are used everyday in life and death situations. Unfortunately, the pressures of cost containment have forced some hospitals to actively pursue vendors who show a promise of lower prices.

Technology is becoming a major selling point for the quality of care provided by medical institutions. While installed cost is an important factor in the selection of a piece of technology, the life cycle costs should also be thoroughly evaluated. The price of the technology should not be the only factor used in making purchasing decisions.

Point 5: *Constantly improve the system of production and service.* The constant improvement of a hospital should be preceded first by a realization of the need for standardization and training in the areas of quality improvement. Continuous improvement is the goal rather than the attainment of a fixed level of quality. This is the key difference between continuous improvement and zero defect. The Deming Cycle (Plan-Do-Check-Act) is based upon the notion that to achieve quality improvement, you must *plan* for it, *do* (implement) it, *check* and analyze the results, and *act* for improvement. This is a never-ending process.

Point 6: *Institute training on the job.* Hospitals emphasize a great deal of training, especially in nursing and medicine. On-the-job (practical) training is a part of the nursing curriculum. Medical students in the third year of medical school are rotated into different clinical specialities for a two year period to gain experience. Even then, they do not receive training on interaction with patients. For nurses, adequate training in patient lifting techniques and reading and interpreting drug labels is sometimes rare.

The health-care field is a humanistic profession, and some hospitals require proper training for the "emotional labor" involved. Not everyone who joins the health-care field is cut out for this type of work. Training is needed for dealing with patients and their visitors who also have to grapple with the emotional burden of ill-health. Some studies have suggested that many nurses and physicians do not have adequate training in using much of the equipment and instruments used in patient care. Lack of training often leads to misuse and abuse of devices, as well as a high rate of calls for help to the biomedical engineering department.

While it is acknowledged that training is essential, it is equally important to emphasize the effectiveness of the training methods used. Training should be aimed principally at eliminating the obstacles to the delivery of good health care as defined by the health-care "customers" and other quality assurance monitoring bodies. Training typically deepens the knowledge a person has about a subject, but if obstacles remain to using that knowledge, it remains untapped.

One of the essential ingredients of continuous improvement, which is often ignored, is an understanding of elementary statistical methods such as means, ranges, and histograms. Hospitals are known to generate a tremendous volume of information daily and managers can use statistical tools to effectively make some sense of the data and enhance decision making.

Point 7: Adopt and institute leadership. Adequate leadership and supervision should focus on being able to help employees achieve excellence in their jobs. One of the goals of a hospital's leadership should be to motivate employees to be a part of the constancy of purpose adopted by the organization. Effective leadership requires knowledge, training, and quality information. Leadership requires knowing when people have special problems and how to improve the work process. Supervisors need to be taught how to design and use the results of patient surveys and how to translate the information obtained into service criteria.

Point 8: *Drive out fear.* Fear inhibits self actualization. One common fear that nurses and other health-care professionals face is the fear of making mistakes. Typical mistakes include administering incorrect dosages of a drug to a patient, giving the wrong drug, inadequate monitoring of patients during drug therapy, ordering the wrong x-rays, etc. Mistakes covered up because an employee is afraid of admitting them can have major implications on quality. Today, many employees still have problems in the area of incident reporting, due to fear of punishment.

Another form of fear often experienced in health-care organizations is the fear of change. With the introduction of DRGs and new concepts, the hospital environment has changed tremendously. One such concept (directed towards cost containment and quality improvement) is clinical information systems. The fear of computers is a prime example of resistance to change. Physicians or top administrators who are experiencing fear can have costly and devastating effects on a health-care organization.

The class distinctions between physicians and nurses, for example, make matters worse. The fear of a domineering head nurse, director of nursing, or physician can put many subordinates in an anxiety-provoking situation. For some nurses, nothing can be more fear-inducing than the thought of an administrator coming off an elevator as the door swings open on a nursing floor.

Interns and residents sometimes have the fear of being perceived by nurses (during their initial introduction to a care delivery routine) as being "dumb" and"incompetent." It is not uncommon to find nurses who yell at the interns, saying something like, "you are the doctor...you should know." Deming (1986) notes that "people on the job cannot work effectively if they dare not enquire into the purpose of the work that they do, and dare not offer suggestions for simplification and improvement of the system." Employees should not be blamed for the problems inherent in the system. The fears of patients are important, too. Mechanisms designed to drive out patient fears like fear of mentally-ill patients, fear of being unable to pay the bill, and fear of certain treatments (chemotherapy) should be developed.

Point 9: *Break down barriers between departments.* The health-care process is multidisciplinary in nature; it draws upon the expertise and support of several departments and people. Some areas in which barriers continue to exist include the following:

• nursing and medical records
• radiology and nurses
• nurses and environmental services (housekeeping)
• physicians, nurses, and pharmacy
• physicians, nurses, pharmacy, and medical records
• admissions, surgery, discharges, and patient control
• clinicians and non-clinicians

Sometimes the senseless desire to protect territory is principally responsible for the barriers. It is not uncommon to find among health-care professionals the perception that one group is inferior to another or that a certain department is made up of "deadbeats." Such perceptions often inhibit the spirit of cooperation among departments or individuals.

Health-care organizations need a model of collaborative practice. According to the National Joint Practice Commission (1977), the definition of collaborative or joint practice in hospitals is "nurses and physicians collaborating as colleagues to provide patient care." H. R. Bradford in a 1989 article notes that the younger physicians and residents perceive the nurse as providing all care, including medical tasks, with no understanding of the nursing process and nursing diagnosis. They do not see the necessity of the nurse and physician collaborating to effect high quality patient care by a combined treatment plan composed of the medical care plan and the nursing care plan. Barriers destroy the spirit of cooperation and lead to lower quality. One way to eliminate barriers is to use cross function teams. A cross function team involves people from various functions and departments. Such a team may consist of employees from the nursing, medicine, pharmacy, laboratory, housekeeping, rehabilitation, record keeping, and information systems departments.

Point 10: *Eliminate slogans, exhortations, and targets for the work force.* Slogans are not very common in health care, although some hospitals continue to rely on them. Some of the common ones are "Nurses make a difference," and "We care." Slogans are no substitute for training. Knowledge of the health-care delivery process, tools, equipment and methods is necessary to help health-care practitioners manage the process. Slogans attempt to shift the responsibility for quality from management to the employees; this is extremely dysfunctional. Only management has the authority to change the system. The implication that these slogans and exhortations can in some miraculous way lead to higher quality is at best ludicrous.

Point 11: *Eliminate numerical quotas for the work force and numerical goals for management.* Work standards and standard costs are not traditionally employed in health-care services. Work sampling technique is more applicable. There are however certain areas in which numerical quotas are utilized. The introduction of DRGs has led to the use of prescribed length of stay values as guidelines or standards for the discharge of patients. The result, in some cases, is that sick patients are sent home—and the incidents of readmission for the same diagnosis are escalating. Also, numerical quotas are used when establishing minimum requirements for maintaining licenses of nurses and doctors. A minimum of 24 to 30 Continuing Education Units is required for nurses every two years, and a minimum of 50 Continuing Medical Education units is required for doctors per year. The tendency in some cases is for nurses and doctors to strive to achieve the minimum requirements and nothing higher.

The following example illustrates the use of numerical quotas in nursing. Suppose that for a two week period, a hospital nursing floor has accumulated 300 patient days. The hospital's finance (administration) department has set a standard of 6.3 hours per patient day for the period. The two figures yield a total of 1890 hours (300 x 6.3). If one Full Time Equivalent (FTE) corresponds to 80 hours (during a two week period), the expected FTE for the nursing floor is 23.6 FTEs (1890 / 80). If the report for that period indicates that the floor actually used 25 FTEs, then that floor is said to be over by almost 2 FTEs, or the equivalent of 160 hours.

The unit is then expected to provide a justification for the difference between the expected FTEs needed and the actual

FTEs used. Such numerical standards can greatly compromise quality of patient care. The emphasis is on working within the FTE requirement guideline rather than on providing quality care. Numerical quotas generate results-oriented rather than performance-oriented behaviors.

Point 12: *Remove barriers that rob people of pride of workmanship. Eliminate the annual rating or merit system.* One of the main barriers that rob people of pride in workmanship is the annual rating or merit system. The performance appraisal system of some health-care organizations can be a major inhibitor to continuing improvement. For example, in certain hospitals, performance evaluation is based on a point system. Pay raises are tied to rating points, especially for nurses. The same process that rates a nurse above average one year might put the nurse below average the next. Dr. Deming suggests that performance appraisal destroys teamwork and focuses on the short term. Many of the perceived differences in people really come from the process, and management is largely to blame. Without an adequate management and control of the process producing the variation, performance will continue to be erratic. The higher up you go in a hospital organization, the more you are likely to fill out your own performance evaluation. The assumption is that you have made your way up the hospital ladder because you are doing well. Performance appraisal systems can inhibit self-actualization and rob people of pride of (workmanship) service.

Point 13: *Institute a vigorous program of education and self-improvement for everyone.* Progressive hospital organizations are beginning to realize that people are the most important assets of an organization. Although many hospitals provide in-house training programs for nurses, radiologists, physical therapists, etc., they generally require employees to sponsor themselves to seminars, and conferences, and also to use their vacation time for it. The in-house training programs sponsored by hospitals are primarily clinical, with little or no attention given to areas such as total quality management, leadership, conflict management, time management, and microcomputer training. There exists a tremendous need for education and training in the technical areas such as drugs, medicines, treatment procedures, and health-care technologies. Health-care organizations need to show a strong commitment to investing in employees. Until this investment is made unselfishly, employees cannot be expected to give their all.

Point 14: Put everyone in the company to work to accomplish the transformation. In order to put everybody in the hospital organization to work to accomplish the transformation, the following key factors are important:

- Management should demonstrate an unequivocal commitment to total quality management. The commitment should be driven by conviction rather than just the need to go along for the sake of it.

- Management should drive out fear and eliminate other inhibitors and barriers to quality improvement in the organization.

- Quality improvement must be preceded first by the education of employees on what quality means and what the needs of the customers are.

- Quality is not a departmental function. It is everyone's business—nurses, physicians, technicians, medical records, fiscal management, pharmacy, among others.

- Quality improvement is a continuous, never-ending process.

- Inspection by the government or any other agency does not mean quality control.

- Quality improvement cannot be accomplished without the total involvement of employees.

Quality According to Feigenbaum

Dr. Armand V. Feigenbaum was the first to introduce the concept of Total Quality Control (TQC). TQC is a concept which makes quality a responsibility to be shared by all the people in an organization. In Japan, the principal responsibility for quality lies with the foremen and the workers, not a quality control department. TQC involves all the functions that pertain to a product or service. One of the underlying views of TQC is that errors or defects should be caught and corrected (if possible) at the source. In the United States, quality cost improvement has kindled research interests among quality experts since Feigenbaum discussed it in his classic book, *Total Quality Control* (1961). Feigenbaum, a consultant, contends that too much is being spent on appraisal and failure costs, and not enough on prevention costs.

Quality According to Ishikawa

Admittedly influenced by the philosophies of Deming, Juran, and Feigenbaum, Kaoru Ishikawa has made significant contributions of his own to the field of quality management. He is credited with developing the concept of quality control circles and their use. He also developed the fishbone diagram (a.k.a. "Ishikawa diagram") which is discussed later in this chapter. Ishikawa notes that in the West, the activity of quality control is generally left to only a few staff specialists—usually in response to a serious problem. Ishikawa notes that by contrast, Japanese managers are totally committed to quality, a commitment that lasts throughout the life of the organization.

Ishikawa has long been considered one of the world's foremost authorities on the subject of quality control. In his book *What is Total Quality Control?* Ishikawa writes about companywide quality control in which all employees, not just quality control specialists, conduct the TQC program. He notes that in the service industry where no manufactured goods are involved, quality assurance means assuring the quality of services rendered. His methods are among the most practical to date. Ishikawa's concept of quality seeks to show the following:

- How to pinpoint the aspects of quality that your customers really want—and are willing to pay for.

- How to go from an inspection-based QC program to a process-oriented one (that includes your customers as part of the process).

- How to use basic statistical tools such as a cause and effect diagrams, Pareto analyses, histograms, etc., to pinpoint the underlying source of errors.

- What steps you must take to root out the primary source of problems so that errors do not recur.

- How to institute voluntary quality control circles to gain more input, understanding, and enthusiasm for your program.

- How to establish and administer a company-wide QC program that includes both vertical and cross-function control.

Ishikawa notes that the practice of quality control seeks to "develop, design, produce and service a quality product which is most economical, most useful, and always satisfactory to the customer." The Japanese-style total quality control has been designated by the term company-wide quality control. According to Ishikawa, "everyone in every division in the company must study, practice, and participate in quality control." In recent years, the company-wide concept has been expanded to include subcontractors, distribution systems, and affiliated companies.

The basic principles of TQC can be summarized as follows:

- Quality is first—not short-term profit.

- Quality is consumer—not producer—oriented. Think from the standpoint of the customer.

- The next process is your customer. Break down the barrier of sectionalism.

- Use facts and data to make presentations and decisions. Utilize statistical methods.

- Respect for humanity is a management philosophy, e.g. full participatory management.

- Management employs cross-functioning.

Quality According to Juran

Dr. Joseph M. Juran, one of the leading authorities in quality control, is a consultant and author and editor of many books including the *Quality Control Handbook* (1974). Juran, like Deming, pioneered the education of the Japanese in the management of quality. Juran's experience suggests that over 80 percent of quality defects are caused by factors controllable by management. Juran stresses the need for management to continually seek improvements using what he defines as the trilogy of quality—planning, control, and improvement.

Quality improvement is a process which begins with identification of an area containing chronic quality problems. Once identified, the need for change and improvement must be conveyed to others to obtain support for change. Next, the alternative solution(s) should be identified and analyzed. The solution(s) with the best potential for continuous improvement should then be implemented. Proper controls for continuous monitoring of the results of the modification should also be in place. It is Juran's view that annual improvement, hands-on management, and training are fundamental to achieving excellence in quality.

Juran's observations about quality health care, as quoted from *Juran on Planning for Quality* (1988) are as follows:

> For years the hospital industry had only the vaguest idea of the extent of errors in the process of giving medication to patients. All hospitals posted rules requiring nurses to report medication errors promptly...however, in many hospitals, the nurses had learned that when they made such reports, they were often subjected to unwarranted blame. Hence they stopped making such reports. In due course, a classic study made by a qualified outsider showed that (1) about seven percent of the medications involved errors, some quite serious, and (2) the bulk of the errors were management-controllable, not worker controllable.

TOTAL SERVICE QUALITY CONTROL (TSQC)

Total service quality control (TSQC) is a business management philosophy, which, when applied to health-care organizations, seeks to provide health-care customers with satisfaction through quality in the services provided. It is a practical approach to quality management based on facts (data), and involves all the employees of an organization (CEO, administrators, nursing, medicine, technical and clinical employees). It is supported by several administrative processes, including quality control teams, policy deployment, cross-functional management, quality in routine activities, and the Deming cycle. Each of these will be discussed below.

Quality Control Teams

Quality control (QC) teams are aimed at providing health-care employees with the opportunity to identify and solve problems. These are trained, organized, and structured groups which identify problems and brainstorm for causes and solutions. The strength of the concept lies in the fact that the problems and solutions are identified by the employees who are directly involved with the problem. The basic premise of QC teams is that nobody knows more about the requirements and problems of a job than the individuals directly responsible for the jobs. Quality control teams benefit the employees through the development of problem-solving skills, the enhancement of communications between employees and management, supervisor-employee cooperation, employee leadership training, and increased employee involvement.

A health-care facility that wants to establish QC teams must first gain an understanding of their mechanics. Many team-development seminars are available today, and it is suggested that management commit training dollars to the education of employees who will be part of a QC team. Management's commitment is a necessary ingredient in the establishment of QC teams.

There are primarily two types of QC teams and they differ according to membership requirements and types of problems tackled. The first type of teams is known as *quality circles. Qual-*

ity circles consist of volunteers who identify problems and work together toward solving them. These employees typically work together on a daily basis and tackle day-to-day work problems. Their primary objective is problem solving using data or facts. Teams of four to twelve people are considered adequate, depending on the size of the work unit. They generally meet between one and two hours per week. Problem solving is typically accomplished through the continuous use of the seven QC tools. Specific applications and design of these tools are presented later in this section.

The second type of team is known as a *task QC team. Task teams* are formed to work on a problem identified by management. Team members are usually appointed and can have diverse backgrounds and positions. The times they spend in meetings is largely a function of the urgency or severity of the problem. Effective team leadership is the key to successful teams in both cases. A task QC team is expected to last for the duration of a given project.

Policy Deployment

Policy deployment is a process in which management works together to focus resources on achieving customer satisfaction for patients and other customers. It relies heavily on the use of task QC teams. Its primary objective is to achieve a breakthrough in areas or issues which are bottlenecked. Policy deployment pursues the achievement of breakthrough by concentrating the efforts and resources of the organization on a few priority issues. Its overall goals include:

- having broad and sustained participation in the development and attainment of an organization's corporate vision.

- achieving cooperation and support in the attainment of long-term, mid-term, and short-term goals of an organization.

- aligning the goals of individual departments in the organization with those of the organization.

- increasing the overall performance of the organization.

Cross-Functional Management

Cross-functional management is defined as all the necessary interdepartmental activities needed to efficiently achieve each of the corporate objectives such as quality, cost, delivery, and so forth, which are basic parameters of sales and profit (Kano 1988). It consists of:

• deploying the strategies for each corporate objective into departmental tactics.

• making each department perform its deployed tactics in its daily management.

• evaluating implemented results from the corporate level.

• taking actions, if necessary.

In hospitals, cross-functional management would involve the management of the interdepartmental strategies for achieving a hospital's corporate objectives. The regular monitoring and management of the results of such strategies is an integral part of cross-functional management. It is not uncommon to find a staff department such as the quality assurance department involved in the coordination of cross functional management activity. On the basis of the functions to be managed, a health-care organization must establish cross-functional committees.

For example, a cross-functional committee on quality may be set up, with the chairman being a senior member of management such as the Chief Medical Officer or the Vice President for Nursing. Committee members are selected from among those who hold top management positions such as division heads, directors, and above. A committee of five to seven members is adequate. It is not essential to draw the committee members only from those who are connected with the specific function. In fact, it is desirable to have one or two persons from other nonrelated divisions of the organization. The committee does not implement quality assurance, nor does it assume day-to-day responsibility for quality assurance. The principal responsi-

bility of the committee is to coordinate interdepartmental activities and allocate resources for quality across all divisions. Its
main function is to coordinate the activities of the various divisions towards the achievement of the corporate goals. The committee typically meets on a monthly basis.

Quality in Routine Activities

Quality in routine activities (QIRA) is a decentralized procedure for controlling and improving daily or routine work. Its
primary objective is to standardize routine activities such as
taking a patient's vital signs or administering routine medication. Also, QIRA seeks to improve standard routine activities
and standardize the gains made. The goals of QIRA are achieved
through quality circle activities. It emphasizes small improvements in the activities carried out voluntarily by staff.

The Deming Cycle (Plan-Do-Check-Act)

The Deming cycle, originally known as the *Shewhart cycle,* named
after its founder W. A. Shewhart, is a method aimed at promot-
ing continuous and never-ending improvement. It was renamed
the Deming cycle by the Japanese in 1950. The cycle (Figure 4-1)
is based upon the premise that to achieve quality improvement,
you must *plan* for it, *do* (implement) it, *check* and analyze the
results, and *act* for improvement. The cycle implies an ongoing
effort to improve all standard routine activities.

Plan. The *plan* begins by first determining what the customers'
needs are (getting well, hot meals, courteous treatment from
staff, cleanliness, accurate diagnosis, state-of-the-art technologies, etc.), setting goals based upon those needs, and planning
how to achieve them. Data concerning customer needs can be
gathered through customer surveys (market research) or direct
interviews. The primary objective is to *plan* how to decrease the
difference between the customer needs and what the process
performs.

Do. In the *do* stage, the *plan* is implemented on a trial basis to see
how it works. The implementation of the *plan* should be done

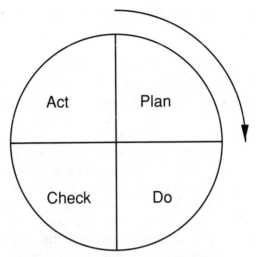

Figure 4-1. The Deming cycle.

on a small scale with a small group of customers. An example would be to raise the food temperature from 130°F to two different higher temperatures of 140°F and 150°F to see how the patients respond. The result of this experiment will become the basis for a permanent plan to meet the expectations of the customers.

Check. During and after the trial run, data must be gathered and analyzed, and the results *checked* to find out what happened: what worked and what did not. The critical question must be "are you closer to your planned goal?"

Act. On the basis of your statistical analysis of the implementation results, you now *act* to ensure that the process improvement is permanent. If in the *check* stage we learned that the patients preferred food temperature of 150°F, then we take proper action to make that change permanent. Education and training should accompany the process of making the change permanent, so that everyone involved understands why the change is needed and how it will be accomplished. Standardization of the gains made is critical to the achievement of quality improvement.

APPLICATION OF QC TOOLS IN TOTAL QUALITY MANAGEMENT

The concept of total quality management is gaining acceptance in the health-care industry, especially as more health-care managers become exposed to the philosophies of Deming, Ishikawa, Crosby, Juran, Feigenbaum, etc. Data are necessary guides for our actions. From data, a health-care organization can learn pertinent facts regarding the causes, extent, scope, and effects of a quality-related problem. Facts provide a consistent basis for action. Continuous improvement begins with an emphasis on the need to teach employees how to identify and analyze quality-related problems, present the suspected causes of the problems, get to their root causes, arrive at the solutions for the problems, and maintain the gains made. The seven QC tools represent an indispensable support system for the success of any TQM program. The tools for organizing and presenting data are:

- checksheets
- graphs
- Pareto analyses
- cause and effect diagrams
- histograms
- scatter diagrams
- control charts

These QC tools are very useful for the "C" in the plan/do/check/act (PDCA) cycle. The remaining part of this chapter primarily explains how to use the seven QC tools in the management and improvement of quality. A framework for continuous quality improvement is presented in Figure 4-2. Before going on to further discussion about the use of the seven QC tools, it is important to examine the meaning of data and procedures for obtaining data.

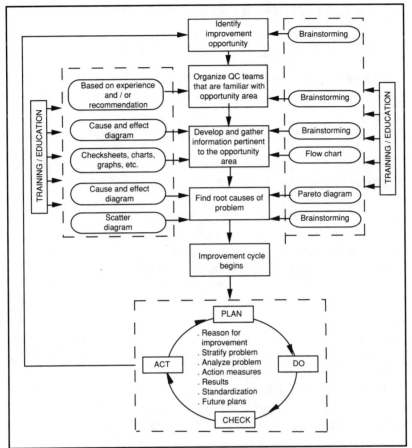

Figure 4-2. Quality improvement (QI) framework.

Data Collection

The process of data collection can be enhanced tremendously by first developing a flow chart of the process. A *flow chart* is a pictorial representation of the various steps of a process, with a view to documenting and better understanding it. It is a widely utilized tool in any type of organization for quality improvement. Its principal advantages are as follows:

- to show the link between activities and identify the next process customer.

• to clarify and document the stages of a process.

• to pinpoint where and when to measure process output.

• to use as a diagnostic tool for troubleshooting problems in the process.

• to facilitate process analyses and improvement.

The most common symbols used in drawing a flowchart can be seen in Figure 4-3.They are used as follows:

• *Ellipse*—used for beginning and ending
• *Rectangle* —used for process activities
• *Diamond*—used for decision points
• *Arrows*—used to indicate direction of flow

Types of Data

Data can be defined as unprocessed (raw) facts, while information is the result of organizing unprocessed facts into something meaningful. For example the number 136 is meaningless by itself, but once we state that it represents the average number of patients' complaints per year in a nursing unit, then it becomes information and meaningful. There are two types of data as explained below:

Attribute or discrete data. These are countable data with pass or fail, go or no go, good or bad, yes or no criterion. The following are examples of attribute data:

• number of misdiagnoses
• number of medication errors
• number of patient-related accidents
• number of phone rings before an answer
• number of patients arriving at an outpatient facility per hour
• frequency of failure of a diagnostic machine
• number of patients' complaints

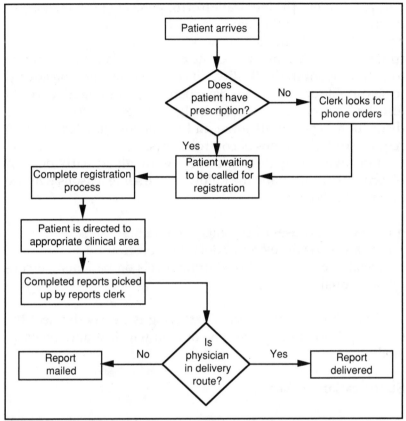

Figure 4-3. A flowchart of an outpatient service.

Variable or continuous data. These are measurable data, reflecting criteria such as how much, how big, and how long. Some examples are:

- response time to patient's call for help
- patients' waiting time
- average food temperature
- ancillary cost for a given patient

The data type can be determined based on the nature of the original data you start with. For example, if your data are medication error percentages, the original data would have been: number of medication errors divided by the total amount of medication administered in that period. Since the original data are discrete, the medication error percentage would also be discrete. If, on the other hand, you are interested in the percentage of time patients spend waiting, the time spent waiting (prior to receiving medical or nursing care) is divided by the total time spent in the facility. Since time is always considered to be variable or continuous data, percent of waiting time would also be variable or continuous. It is necessary to make the distinction between attribute and variable data because each requires different types of control charts.

Effective data gathering must begin with a clearly defined objective. In health care, the following are some reasons why we might collect data:

- to study the causes of patients' complaints
- to analyze the problems of delays in test results
- to evaluate the impact of staffing levels on patients' perception of quality of care

Once the objective of data gathering is clearly defined, the next step is to identify the type of data which should be gathered.

Stratification of Data

Suppose, for example, that there is a problem involving high incidence of medication errors. Data collection must be directed at individual nurses or pharmacists, rather than sampling the group or team on duty. If comparing one nurse against the other reveals a clear difference, then a remedial action can be taken to correct the problem. The process of breaking down the group (total area of concern) into smaller, related subgroups is called *stratification*. Stratification of information makes it easier to do a more precise analysis of it. Stratification can also be a powerful tool in quantifying the root cause of a problem. Other ways to fully understand the types of data needed would be to stratify by shift, nursing skill levels, patient age groups or gender, nursing unit, diagnoses, length of stay, etc.

The process of data collection can be very challenging when you want to investigate the relationship between two variables such as the number of patients' complaints regarding the staff's failure to answer call lights promptly and patient acuity levels. Since this involves studying the relationship between the values of two characteristics, the data have to be available in pairs—for each nursing unit. Once the data are gathered in pairs, they can be analyzed using a scatter diagram which is explained later in this chapter.

RELIABILITY OF DATA

The reliability of data is as important as the data collection process itself. Even if the correct type of data has been collected, a wrong judgment or decision will be made if the data is unreliable. Proper care should be taken to ensure that there are no missing data or incorrect entries made. Adequate training and information on the importance of accurate and reliable data are essential in ensuring the reliability of data. Intermediate handling of data should be discouraged and direct and immediate entry (via computer) should be emphasized.

Once it has been decided that certain types of data are necessary, the next step is to decide the proper ways to record them. It is important to arrange data systematically to facilitate analysis and subsequent processing. It is extremely important to clearly identify the origin of the data. This makes verification possible. Other useful information to be recorded along with the data are the days of the week on which data are based, names or codes of individuals involved in the activities, time of the day, nursing units, shifts, and diagnoses.

Since most data are often used later to compute statistics such as means, frequency, ranges, etc., it is better to record them in a manner which will facilitate these computations. If it is determined that data will be collected on a continuous basis, then standard recording forms should be designed before hand.

Checksheets

A checksheet is a form used for the purpose of collecting data systematically by making simple marks under the appropriate categories. See Figures 4-4 to 4-6 for examples. A checksheet makes it possible to gather data easily into categories by recording marks that show visible patterns. The three main purposes of a checksheet are:

1. to simplify the process of data gathering.
2. to organize data for easy use.
3. to eliminate rehandling of data and recording errors.

A Case Example

Suppose a hospital is concerned about the number of complaints in the following areas:

- increased number of Caesarean section births
- poor food services
- noise levels

SAMPLE CHECKSHEET

Date

Type of Complaint Caesarean section

Nursing Unit

Remarks

Analyst

Total no. of records 300

Types of causes	Checks	Frequency
Cephalo-Pelvic disproportion	卌 卌 卌 卌	20
Infants in breech positions	卌 III	8
Fetal distress	卌 II	7
Previous births by C-section	卌 I	6
Other causes	卌 IIII	9
	Total	50

Figure 4-4. A checksheet for Caesarean section.

SAMPLE CHECKSHEET

Date(s) <u>1/89 - 6/89</u>

Type of Complaint <u>Noise</u>

Nursing Unit _____

Remarks _____

Analyst _____

	Unit Name	Checks	Frequency
UNIT-BASED	Unit #A	卌 卌 l	11
	Unit #B	卌 l	6
	Unit #C	lll	3
	- - -	- - -	- -
	Unit #D	卌	5

Figure 4-5. A checksheet for number of unit-based complaints.

- cleanliness (lack of)
- failure to answer call lights promptly

In order to better understand the type of data to be collected, we must first categorize these issues as hospital-based or unit-based as shown in Table 4-1.

Table 4-1. Classification of patients' complaints.

Hospital-based	Nursing unit-based
• Poor food services	• Noise
• Cleanliness (lack of)	• Failure to answer call light promptly
• Caesarean-section births	

SAMPLE CHECKSHEET

Date(s) <u>1/89 - 6/89</u>

Type of Complaint <u>Cleanliness (lack of)</u>

Nursing Unit _____

Remarks _____

Analyst _____

	Days	Checks	Frequency
	Day 1	III	3
	Day 2	~~IIII~~ II	7
HOSPITAL-WIDE	**Day 3**	II	2
	- - -	- - -	- -
	Day n	~~IIII~~	5

Figure 4-6. A checksheet for number of hospital-wide complaints.

Graphs

Graphs are visual displays of quantitative data over time. With the aid of graphs, it is easy to expose any patterns or trends in the data. Graphs are communication tools that enhance our understanding and interpretation of complex phenomena. The most common graph form is a line graph (Figure 4-7). The characteristics of a good graph are:

• All graphs should have a title which shows the information being presented.
• The scale of a graph should be selected to accommodate potential variable changes.

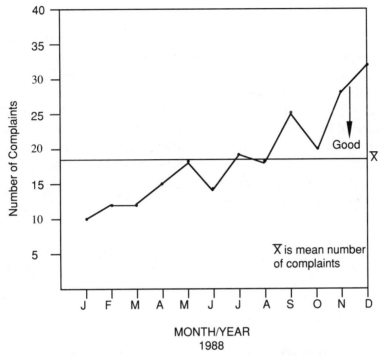

Figure 4-7. A line graph showing patient complaints about food temperature. Compiled from patient services log sheets.

• The y- and x-axes of a graph should be properly labeled to reflect the categories of data. For example, in the case of a line graph, the x-axis represents the measurement intervals, usually units of time, and the y-axis is the variable or factor being measured.

• If there is a "good" direction in the line graph (up or down), this should be indicated with an arrow. This becomes obvious once the points are plotted and connected.

• Every graph should indicate data source, the name of the person who gathered the data, date (and time if necessary) when data was collected, and how the data was collected. Suppose that the information below represents complaints over food and temperature at a local hospital. The values are then plotted on a line graph (see Figure 4-7).

Pareto Analysis

In health care, as in many other fields, we are often confronted by quality-related problems that must first be identified, and then eliminated. Pareto analysis is a way of organizing data to show the *vital few* causes of the problem in contrast to the *trivial many*. An example is the "80-20 rule," which implies that 80 percent of the problems are caused by 20 percent of the causes.

In 1897, Vilfredo Pareto, an Italian economist presented a formula which shows unevenness in income distribution. In 1907, M.C. Lorenz, an American economist also expressed a similar theory diagrammatically. Both Pareto and Lorenz noted that by far the largest share of the income or wealth was in the hands of a small number of people. J. M. Juran applied this concept to quality problems in order to classify them into the *vital few* and the *trivial many*, and named this procedure, Pareto Analysis.

Steps in Making Pareto Diagrams

Step 1. Identify what problems are to be investigated and decide how to collect the data. Pareto works best for zero-based types of data, such as number of complaints or number of mistakes; the ideal situation is to reduce it to zero.

Step 2. Classify the data by categories such as type of complaints, nursing units, shifts, diagnosis related groups, patients, etc.

Step 3. If possible, you may further stratify weekly data into weekdays and weekends, and classify each day by shift, such as morning, day, and night shifts. This is called a *second level Pareto.*

A Case Example
To illustrate the remaining steps, consider the case of a local hospital whose complaint rate during the period 6/89 - 12/89 is given as follows :

Nursing Unit	Number of Complaints
A	12
B	22
C	61
D	5
E	10

Suppose unit C is selected for further study due to its comparatively high rate of complaints.

Step 4. Make a Pareto diagram data sheet listing the types of complaints, their respective totals, cumulative totals, percentage of overall total, and cumulative percentages as shown below in Table 4-2.

Step 5. Arrange the types of complaints in descending order of quantity, and complete the rest of the data sheet. Note: All complaints should be categorized, but the complaints that occur infrequently can be lumped into the "others" category and should be placed in the last line. This is because it is composed of a group of complaints, each of which is smaller than the smallest complaint listed individually. Rule of thumb: if "others" is more than 50 percent of the biggest value, break it out to sub causes.

Step 6. Make the Pareto graph by drawing two vertical axes and a horizontal axis. Mark the left-hand vertical axis with a scale from 0 to the overall total (which in our case is 61). Mark the right-hand vertical axis with a scale from 0% to 100%. Divide the horizontal axis into the number of complaint types.

Step 7. Construct the bar diagram.

Step 8. Draw the cumulative curve (Pareto curve). Mark the cumulative points above the right-hand intervals of each complaint type, and connect the points by a solid line as shown in Figure 4-8.

Table 4-2. Data sheet for Pareto diagram.

Types of Complaints for Nursing Unit C	Number of Complaints	Cumulative Total	Percent of Overall Total	Cumulative Percent
Poor food services	33	33	54	54
Rudeness of staff	12	45	20	74
Noise	4	49	7	81
Inadequate explanations	2	51	3	84
Others	10	61	16	100
Total	61	--	100	--

Step 9. Check your graph for the Pareto pattern; a "flat" pattern—categories with similar percentages—indicates the need for different stratification of the data. A "flat" Pareto is one in which there is no distinct category of "vital flow" and "trivial many." Each block of "cause" is not distinctly different from the other.

Note: The above type of Pareto diagram is known as *Pareto diagram by phenomena.* The next step is to go into *poor food services,* which in this case represents the vital few, and do a Pareto diagram by causes.

Cause and Effect Diagrams (Ishikawa or "Fishbone Diagram")

A cause and effect diagram shows the relationship between a quality characteristic and factors. It is used primarily to analyze a problem by narrowing it down to a few possible root causes so that they can be investigated and selectively verified, as depicted in Figure 4-9.

In 1953, Professor Kaoru Ishikawa of the University of Tokyo, Japan, applied the concept of cause and effect to a quality problem. The Ishikawa diagram or "fishbone diagram" (since it can look like the skeleton of a fish) is in the form of a chart composed of lines and words designed to represent a meaningful relationship between an effect and its causes. One of the supportive techniques for making a cause and effect diagram is brainstorming.

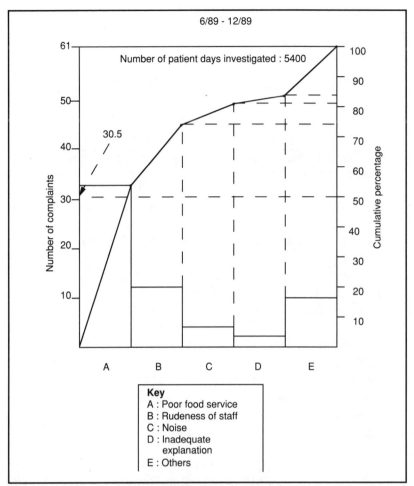

Figure 4-8. Pareto diagram by types of complaints.

Brainstorming is a technique used to generate ideas and identify issues and problem areas. It emphasizes the quantity of ideas rather than the quality. In the context of TQC, brainstorming is used to tap the creative thinking of quality improvement team members. There are three phases in the brainstorming technique: the *creation phase,* the *refinement phase,* and the *assessment phase.*

The creation phase. The team leader begins this phase by first stating the topic to be brainstormed and going over the rules of brainstorming as follows:

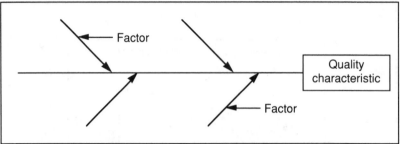

Figure 4-9. Schematic of a cause and effect diagram showing factor and quality characteristics.

- Each group member takes a turn, in sequence, to supply one idea at a time.
- The creation phase continues until all ideas have been exhausted.
- Criticism or discussion on any idea is not permitted.
- It is acceptable for anyone to pass (if he/she has no new idea).
- It is acceptable to build on the ideas of others.

The topic to be brainstormed must be stated clearly and precisely. A recorder should be selected from within the group to record the ideas generated. Ideas should be recorded in a manner that will make them visible to all team members. One of the most common forms of recording the ideas is to print them on flip charts in large handwriting and display on the walls.

The refinement phase. During this phase of brainstorming, members of the team would go over the compiled list of ideas to make sure that all participants understand all the items. No discussion or criticism of ideas should be entertained in this phase.

The assessment phase. During the assessment phase, the team goes over the list to eliminate duplications and issues that are not germane to the topic. Teams may use a structured series of votes to help reduce the list of ideas to a manageable size.

Procedures for Making a Cause and Effect Diagram

Step 1. Select a problem, which in our example is the high rate of complaints about food services. This problem is in essence, the effect or quality characteristic.

Step 2. Using the brainstorming technique (working with a group of 4 to 12 people), develop a list of possible causes of the problem.

Step 3. Group all the causes into major categories (primary causes). A common grouping is by causes related to manpower, methods, materials, machinery, and environment.

Step 4. Draw the diagram by writing the problem (effect) clearly in a box on the right-hand side of the paper. Draw in the "backbone," which is a horizontal line running from left to right and touching the effect box with an arrowhead. Build the diagram by linking the brainstormed causes under the appropriate categories. Write the causes (secondary causes) which affect the primary causes (the major categories), and also tertiary causes which affect the secondary causes. Lines should flow toward the "effect" and touch with arrowheads.

Step 5. Continue to refine categories as well as the relationships among the primary, secondary, and tertiary causes by constantly asking:

• What causes this condition?
• Why does the condition exist?
• Is it a cause or a symptom?

The process of refinement must continue until the causes stated are specific enough to verify and act upon. (See Figure 4-10 for the cause and effect diagram for our food services example). Note also that if the causes you have identified are not amenable to corrective action, then the problem will not be solved. If improvements are to be implemented, the selected causes must be broken down to the level at which corrective action is feasible, otherwise simply itemizing the root causes will be an investment in futility.

Step 6. Through the use of data, rank the causes identified according to importance. This should not be done solely on the basis of opinions. Once a particular cause has been eliminated, it should be deleted and the cause and effect diagram should be updated. You may also discover other new causes to be added to the diagram. A cause and effect diagram should be continuously updated while it is being used.

A second level cause and effect diagram may also be generated from our food services example. Suppose that after further examination of the patient services log sheet, it is determined that the most important cause of food services related complaints is food temperature. A second level cause and effect diagram can then be drawn as shown in Figure 4-11.

Histograms

A histogram is used to display continuous data (measurable data such as time) as opposed to discrete data (countable data, such as number of complaints). By organizing data on a histogram, we gain a better understanding of the distribution of the data. The following example illustrates the use of histograms:

A Case Example
Suppose that a local hospital nursing unit collected the following data about the time it takes nurses to respond to call lights during a one week period.

Time to Respond to Patients' Call Lights (in seconds)
(Evening Shift)

328	292	399	310	87	360
320	608	302	325	391	368
462	512	227	127	407	43
247	338	560	362	487	309
882	335	843	348	335	512
228	960	308	569	359	590
69	577	422	632	362	302
365	502	559	423	403	618
720	387	301	701	512	374
308	344	340	399	312	342

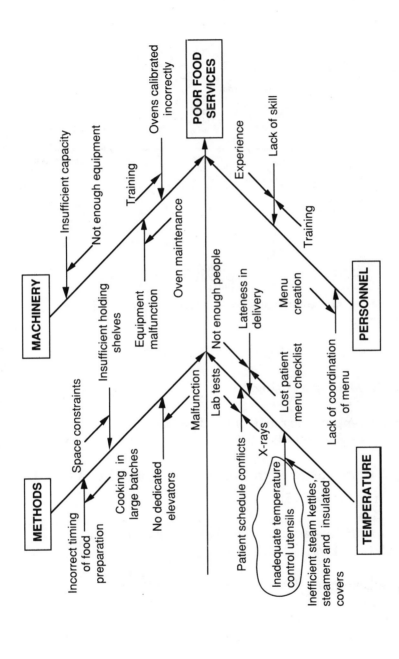

Figure 4-10. An example of a cause and effect diagram for food services complaints.

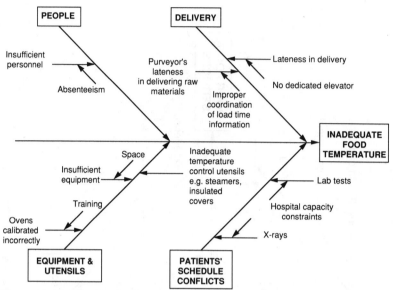

Figure 4-11. An example of a cause and effect diagram for food temperature.

Steps in Making a Histogram

Step 1. Compute the range of the data (R)
$$R = X_{max} - X_{min} = 960 - 43 = 917$$

Step 2. Compute the approximate number of classes (C)
$$C = \sqrt{n} = \sqrt{60} = 7.75$$

Step 3. Compute approximate class width (W)
$$W = R/C = 917/7.75 = 118.32$$

Step 4. Determine the unit of measurement (m)
$$m = 1$$

Step 5. Round off the class width (W) and number of classes (C)
$$W = 118$$
$$C = 8$$

Step 6. Compute the lower boundary of the first class
$L_1 = X_{min} - (m/2) = 43 - (1/2) = 42.5$

Step 7. Determine the lower boundaries of the remaining classes
$L_2 = 42.5 + 118 = 160.5$
$L_3 = 160.5 + 118 = 278.5$
$L_4 = 278.5 + 118 = 396.5$
$L_5 = 396.5 + 118 = 514.5$
$L_6 = 514.5 + 118 = 632.5$
$L_7 = 632.5 + 118 = 750.5$
$L_8 = 750.5 + 118 = 868.5$
$L_9 = 868.5 + 118 = 986.5$

Step 8. Construct a frequency table of the data (Table 4-3).

Step 9. Construct a histogram for the frequency table (see Figure 4-12).

Scatter Diagram

A scatter diagram is a technique for studying the relationship between two variables factors (see Figure 4-13).

A scatter diagram represents a plot of pairs of data involving two variables. A scatter diagram will reveal any existing patterns in the data and will also show the strength of the relationship between both variables. Although the technique is often used for discrete data (countable data), its correct application is when the two variables are continuous data (measurable data).

Examples of possible areas of application for a scatter diagram include the following:

• To study the relationship between food temperature upon arrival to patient and speed of delivery in minutes (the amount of time between the food being removed from the oven and the patient receiving it).

• To examine the relationship between patient waiting time after pushing the call button and the time of day.

Table 4-3. Frequency table for a histogram.

Frequency Table		
Class Interval	**Tally**	**Frequency**
42.5-160.5	IIII	4
160.5-278.5	III	3
278.5-396.5	HHH HHH HHH HHH III	23
396.5-514.5	HHH HHH II	12
514.5-632.5	HHH III	8
632.5-750.5	II	2
750.5-868.8	I	1
868.5-986.5	II	2

- To investigate the relationship between hours spent training new nurses and the hours spent correcting patient chart errors.

Perhaps the most important application of a scatter diagram lies in its use to verify the relationship between the factor that you suspect is the most important and the corresponding quality characteristics.

How to Construct a Scatter Diagram

Step 1. Collect paired data (x,y) and arrange them in a data table. As a general rule, a minimum of 30 pairs of data is desirable. The x values represent the *independent* variables (cause), while the y values represent the *dependent* variables (quality characteristic or another factor). Select the horizontal axis as the x-axis and the vertical as the y-axis.

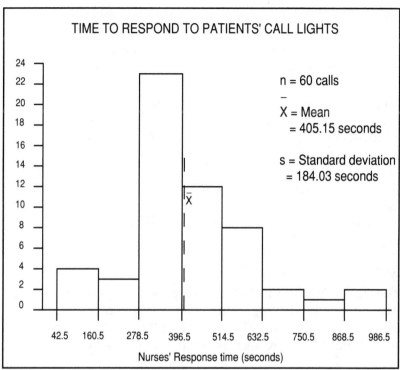

Figure 4-12. A histogram showing response time to patients' call lights.

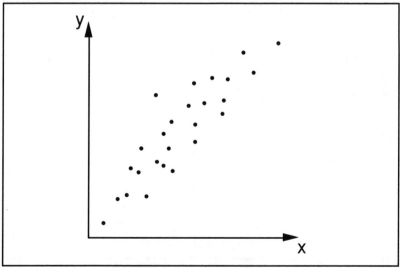

Figure 4-13. An example of a scatter diagram.

Step 2. Identify the maximum and minimum values for both the x and y scales. The scales of the horizontal and vertical axes should be selected in such a way that both lengths would be approximately equal.

Step 3. Plot the pairs of (x,y) data. When the same data values exist for different observations, distinguish these points either by drawing a circle around each one or by plotting the second point as close as possible to the first.

Step 4. Complete the diagram by adding all other pertinent information such as diagram title, number of data points, time interval, labels for x- and y-axes, and the name of the diagram preparer.

A Case Example
The data presented in Table 4-4 represents information on actual patient food temperature and the speed of the delivery (measured as the time taken to deliver the tray to the patient). A scatter diagram of the data is given in Figure 4-14.

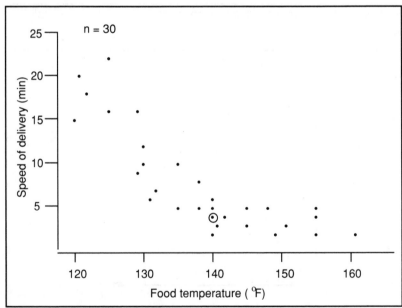

Figure 4-14. Scatter diagram of speed of delivery and food temperature.

Table 4-4. Data for case example.

Item Number	Food Temperature (°F)	Speed of Delivery (min)
1	140	2
2	135	5
3	131	6
4	130	10
5	141	3
6	120	15
7	121	20
8	140	4
9	129	16
10	138	5
11	140	5
12	145	3
13	125	22
14	151	3
15	132	7
16	145	5
17	148	5
18	122	18
19	135	10
20	129	9
21	149	2
22	142	4
23	140	4
24	140	6
25	155	5
26	125	16
27	130	12
28	138	8
29	161	2
30	155	3

How to Interpret Scatter Diagrams

When the relationship between two variables can be described by a straight line, it is said to be a linear relationship. There are also non-linear relationships, however, that subject will not be covered in this book. Figure 4-15 illustrates how to interpret scatter diagrams.

How to Determine Correlation Coefficient (r)

Scatter diagrams can usually be interpreted visually; however, if more preciseness is desired, the correlation coefficient (r) can be calculated in the following manner:

$$r = \frac{n \operatorname{sum}(xy) - \operatorname{sum}(x)\operatorname{sum}(y)}{\sqrt{\left[n \operatorname{sum}(x^2) - (\operatorname{sum} x)^2\right]\left[n \operatorname{sum}(y)^2 - (\operatorname{sum} y)^2\right]}}$$

where
n = sample size
y = dependent variable (speed of delivery) and quality characteristic
x = independent variable (food temperature) and factor
r = coefficient of correlation; where r is between -1 and +1. Perfect negative correlation is indicated by -1, and +1 indicates perfect positive correlation. At a correlation coefficient of +1 or -1, all of the data points will lie exactly on a straight line.

Table 4-5 shows how to arrange the data to facilitate the computation of correlation coefficient *r*.

$$r = \frac{25(25,473) - (194)(3,423)}{\sqrt{\left[25(470,837) - (3,423)^2\right]\left[25(2,324) - (194)^2\right]}}$$

$$r = \frac{-27,237}{\sqrt{(53,996)(20,464)}}$$

r = -27,237/33,241

r = -0.82

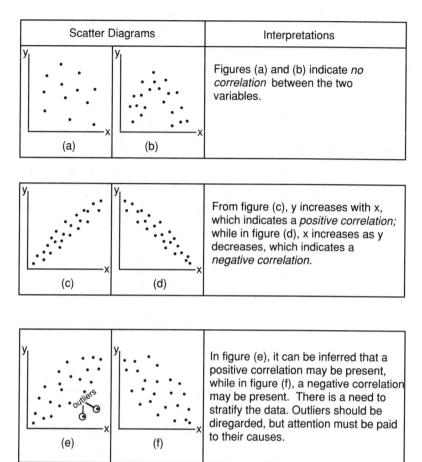

Figure 4-15. Interpretation of scatter diagrams.

Note: The value of -0.82 represents a negative correlation between food temperature and speed of delivery.

An Outpatient Case Example

The following example was developed by Erin M. Gately and Jeffrey D. Tomaszewski of the University of Miami in 1989.

The outpatient clinic of a local hospital serves approximately 200 patients per day, Monday through Friday, and 75 patients on Saturday. The hours of operation are 6:00 a.m. to 6:00 p.m. Monday through Friday and 7:00 a.m. to 1:00 p.m. on Saturday. The clinic is staffed by a team of 21 employees. Of this, ten are responsible for actual registration, four are patient escorts, three

Table 4-5. Data arrangement for correlation computation.

Item No.	Speed of Delivery (minutes) Y	Food Temperature X (°F)	Y^2	X^2	XY
1	2	140	4	19600	280
2	5	135	25	18225	675
3	6	131	36	17161	786
4	10	130	100	16900	1300
5	3	141	9	19881	423
6	15	120	225	14400	1800
7	20	121	400	14641	2420
8	4	140	16	19600	560
9	16	129	256	16641	2064
10	5	138	25	19044	690
11	5	140	25	19600	700
12	3	145	9	21025	435
13	22	125	484	15625	2750
14	3	151	9	22801	453
15	7	132	49	17424	924
16	5	145	25	21025	725
17	5	148	25	21904	740
18	18	122	324	14884	2196
19	10	135	100	18225	1350
20	9	129	81	16641	1161
21	2	149	4	22201	298
22	4	142	16	20164	568
23	4	140	16	19600	560
24	6	140	36	19600	840
25	5	155	25	24025	775
Total	194	3,423	2,324	470,837	25,473

are supervisors, one is a registration clerk, one is in charge of scheduling, one works as a telephone operator, and one person is in charge of special projects.

The hospital's outpatient clinic handles, among other things, the processing of patients through various tests such as blood tests, urinalysis, etc. The process begins when the physician requests a certain procedure. As Figure 4-16 illustrates, the doctor's office may schedule the appointment, the patient may schedule it, or the patient may elect to walk in at his or her leisure. When scheduling receives a phone call, the operator decides whether or not the examination needs to be scheduled. In case it does not need to be scheduled, the order is recorded and the patient can come in at any time. If the exam must be scheduled, an appointment is made and the patient is preregistered. After the patient arrives, the check-in clerk asks the patient for the prescription. If the patient does not have the prescription, the clerk proceeds to locate the phone order placed by the doctor. At this point the patient waits to be called for registration. Once called, the registration process begins. Upon completion of registration, the patient is directed to the appropriate clinical area. Completed reports are then picked up by the reports clerk and delivered by hand or mailed to the physician.

The Problem

Patients receiving care from the outpatient clinic have complained of excessive waiting prior to being registered. Management is aware that the registration process takes too long and has determined that a waiting time of more than 20 minutes in the queue is unacceptable. The tools of TQC can be applied to study and improve the quality of the service provided by the clinic by reducing the waiting times and delays.

Data Collection and Analysis

An initial study of the number of patients received per day reveals the following information presented in Table 4-6. Figure 4-17 shows a column graph indicating the number of patients received by day of the week. Tables 4-7a and 4-7b present

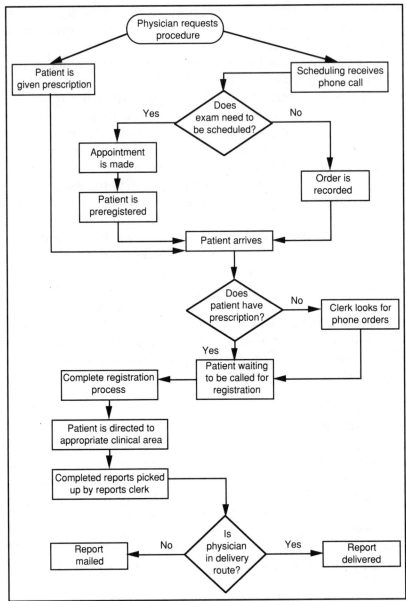

Figure 4-16. A flowchart of an outpatient service.

information on the number of patients received by day and by time of day. This information is helpful to pindown the scope and source of problems. A column graph on the information is presented in Figure 4-18.

Table 4-6. Average number of patients per day of the week.

Days	Patients Received	Cumulative Total	Percent	Cumulative Percent
Monday	200	200	22.3	22.3
Tuesday	199	399	22.2	44.5
Wednesday	178	577	19.9	64.4
Thursday	165	742	18.4	82.8
Friday	154	896	17.2	100.0

Later in this project, it was determined that perhaps a distinction should be made between patients with appointments and those without appointments. However, no significant differences were observed in waiting times (Table 4-8). Suppose that management has determined that an average waiting time of 20 minutes or less is acceptable. Table 4-9 gives the pertinent data and the resulting column graph is shown in Figure 4-19.

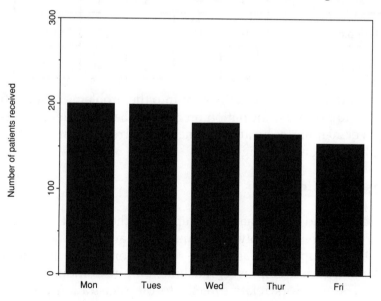

Figure 4-17. Number of patients by day.

Table 4-7a. Average number of patients received.

Time	Mon	Tue	Wed	Thur	Fri	Average
6 - 7 a.m.	2	6	3	4	5	4.0
7 - 8 a.m.	20	26	19	24	16	21.0
8 - 9 a.m.	22	25	26	25	24	24.4
9 - 10 a.m.	25	28	30	18	15	23.2
10 - 11 a.m.	20	18	17	13	21	17.8
11 - 12 noon	18	15	14	11	15	14.6
12 - 1 p.m.	15	13	12	14	11	13.0
1 - 2 p.m.	17	19	13	10	12	14.2
2 - 3 p.m.	18	16	14	17	12	15.4
3 - 4 p.m.	15	14	14	15	14	14.4
4 - 5 p.m.	14	14	12	12	8	12.0
5 - 6 p.m.	15	7	7	5	4	7.6

In order to gain further insight into the problem, Table 4-10 is used to present information on the number of patients waiting over 20 minutes by arrival time. The corresponding column graph is presented in Figure 4-20.

Cause and Effect

The cause and effect diagrams represent the output of brainstorming exercises involving the managers and employees. Figure 4-21 groups the reasons for registration delays into four major categories: employee, machine, administration, and patient. These factors relate directly to the registration process, whereas Figure 4-22 is related to the amount of time taken

Table 4-7b. Average number of patients received and cumulative percentages.

Time	Average	Cumulative Average	Percent	Cumulative Percent
8 - 9 a.m.	24.4	24.4	13.4	13.4
9 - 10 a.m.	23.2	47.6	12.8	26.2
7 - 8 a.m.	21.0	68.6	11.6	37.8
10 - 11 a.m.	17.8	86.4	9.8	47.6
2 - 3 p.m.	15.4	101.8	8.5	56.1
11 - 12 noon	14.6	116.4	8.0	64.1
3 - 4 p.m.	14.4	130.8	7.9	72.0
1 - 2 p.m.	14.2	145.0	7.8	79.8
12 - 1 p.m.	13.0	158.0	7.2	87.0
4 - 5 p.m.	12.0	170.0	6.6	93.6
5 - 6 p.m.	7.6	177.6	4.2	97.8
6 - 7 a.m.	4.0	181.6	2.2	100.0

before calling the patient to be registered. Table 4-11 represents a list of the reasons for the delays in the registration process and the frequency of occurrence. The corresponding Pareto diagram is presented in Figure 4-23.

Summary of Results

- 55% of delays in registration are caused by:
    - Inadequate staffing
    - Need to look up test in book
    - Failure by doctors to include diagnosis

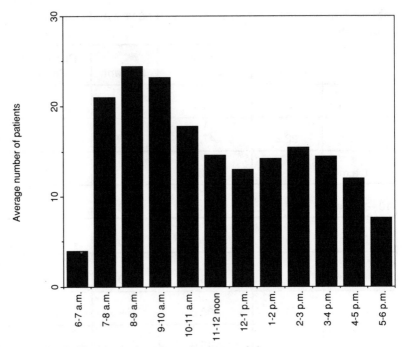

Figure 4-18. Number of patients by hour of day.

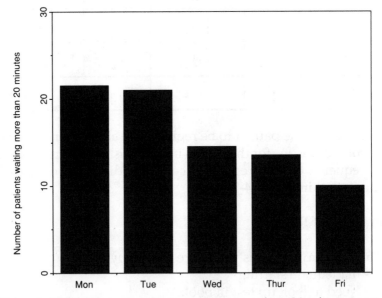

Figure 4-19. Number of patients waiting more than 20 minutes per day.

Table 4-8. Average waiting times for patients with and without appointments.

Days	Avg. No. of Patients with Appointments	Avg. Waiting Time/ Patient (min)	Avg. No. of Patients without Appointments	Avg. Waiting Time/ Patient (min)	Combined Avg. Waiting Time/ Patient
Monday	104	10.26	96	10.09	10.18
Tuesday	99	10.80	104	10.51	10.66
Wednesday	92	9.73	87	9.82	9.78
Thursday	87	8.89	79	8.91	8.90
Friday	94	7.82	76	9.41	8.62

- Approximately 62% of the patients waiting over 20 minutes do so between the hours of 7 a.m. to 10 a.m. About 80% of the patients waiting over 20 minutes do so between 7 a.m. and 11 a.m.

- Approximately 53% of the patients waiting over 20 minutes do so on Mondays and Tuesdays.

- There is no significant difference in waiting time between patients with appointments and those without appointments.

Table 4-9. Number of patients waiting more than 20 minutes per day.

Days	Avg. No. of Patients Waiting	Cumulative Total	Percent	Cumulative Percent
Monday	21.5	21.5	26.7	26.7
Tuesday	21.0	42.5	26.0	52.7
Wednesday	14.5	57.0	18.0	70.7
Thursday	13.5	70.5	16.8	87.5
Friday	10.0	80.5	12.5	100.0

Table 4-10. Number of patients waiting over 20 minutes by arrival time.

Hour	No. >20 min.	Cumulative Total	Percent	Cumulative Percent
8 - 9 a.m.	39	39	26.9	26.9
9 - 10 a.m.	28	67	19.3	46.2
7 - 8 a.m.	22	89	15.2	61.4
2 - 3 p.m.	15	104	10.3	71.7
10 - 11 a.m.	12	116	8.2	79.9
1 - 2 p.m.	12	128	8.2	88.1
12 - 1 p.m.	9	137	6.1	94.2
3 - 4 p.m.	5	142	3.4	97.6
11 - 12 noon	2	144	1.4	99.0
4 - 5 p.m.	1	145	1.0	100.0
6 - 7 a.m.	0	145	0.0	100.0
5 - 6 p.m.	0	145	0.0	100.0

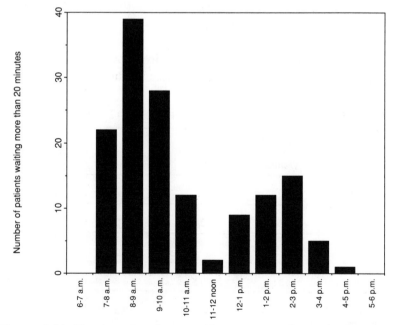

Figure 4-20. Number of patients waiting over 20 minutes by hour.

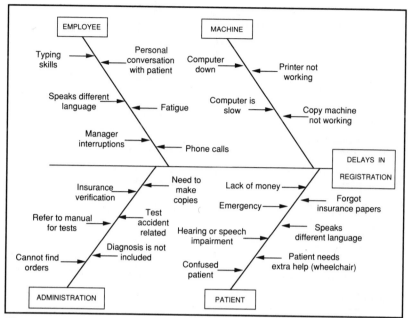

Figure 4-21. Cause and effect diagram for delays in registration (actual registration).

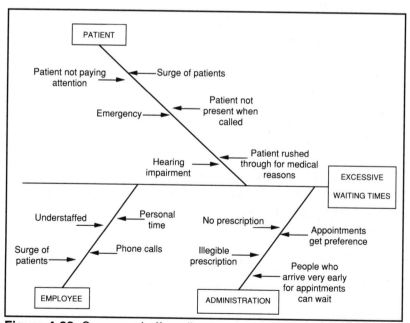

Figure 4-22. Cause and effect diagram for excessive waiting times before registration.

Table 4-11. Delays in the registration process.

Reason for Delay	Percentage Occurrence	Cumulative Percentage
Inadequate staffing	30	30
Need to look up test in book	15	45
Doctors diagnosis not included	10	55
Confused or disoriented patient	10	65
Phone call while not with patient	10	75
Phone call while with patient	9	84
Patient forgot insurance papers	5	89
Patient accompanied by child	5	94
Test is accident related	5	99

- Approximately 50% of the patients received arrive between 7 a.m. and 11 a.m., with the largest group arriving between 8 a.m. and 9 a.m.

- Approximately 45% of the patients handled come in on Mondays and Tuesdays.

The process of continuous improvement is by no means complete. Efforts must now be directed at eliminating the root causes of the problems. Some improvement actions that can be taken include:

- Hiring an additional registrar to handle peak demand periods. This could be an an expensive manpower fix.

- Optimizing the scheduling process to compliment the work load. It should be noted that the system cannot be optimized if

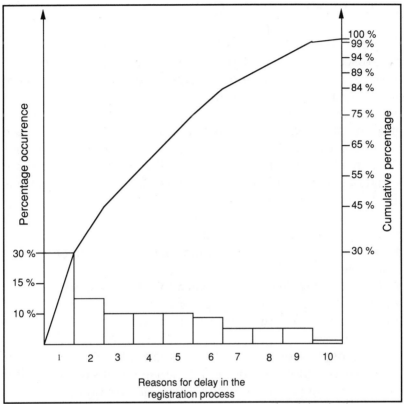

Figure 4-23. Pareto diagram showing reasons for delay in the registration process.

the system is not stable. The use of a control chart might therefore be necessary.

- Developing a standard code of abbreviations for tests so that doctors and lab technicians can refer to them by the same name. This will cut down on the time it takes to look up the proper names of the tests.

- Developing an efficient procedure for having doctors include the diagnosis in the prescription.

- Calling the patient a day before to remind him/her to bring appropriate insurance papers, prescription, etc., for ease of processing.

Control Charts

Before explaining the concept of control charts, it is important to first discuss the concept of process variations. All processes have some form of variation inherent in them as variations are simply unavoidable. For example, the proportion of medication or billing errors will vary from one day to another. A conscious effort must be made to control and reduce variations. There are two types of variations: variations due to *common causes* and those due to *special causes*. Variations due to common causes are variations that are inherent in a process. Examples of variations due to common causes are:

• poor lighting in a nursing unit
• inadequate working environment, such as noise, poor ventilation, etc.
• failure to provide feedback to health-care personnel
• out-of-order diagnostic equipment
• poorly designed clinical information system

Employees should not be held responsible for problems that are due to common variations. It is management's responsibility to do something about common causes of variations.

Variations that are due to special causes are variations that fall outside the system. Special cause variations are avoidable and should not be overlooked. Examples include cases caused by not following certain prescribed standards or the application of improper standards. Special causes are also largely due to differences among workers, methods, and machines. In both cases, variations should be identified and managed. When variations are due to special causes, it implies the presence of certain meaningful factors that should be investigated.

Control charts are graphic aids for detecting process output variations due to special causes. A control chart consists of a central line (based on the average), an upper control limit and a lower control limit. The limits are drawn at a calculated distance above and below the central line. Figure 4-24 depicts what a control chart looks like.

When points fall outside the control limits, have a run of seven or more above or below the center line, have a run of

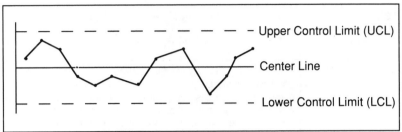

Figure 4-24. An example of a control chart.

seven or more up or down, or exhibit other non-random patterns, we say that the process is out-of-control.

Types of Control Charts

The types of control charts available as well as the types of data for which they can be used are summarized in Table 4-12. Table 4-13 gives a description of each of the charts.

A Case Example
An inspection of a hospital's patient accounting records reveals the information in Table 4-14 regarding billing errors.

Table 4-12. Types of control charts and corresponding data types.

Type of Chart	Data Type
$\bar{X}$-R Chart (average value and range)	Variable data (continuous value)
X Chart (measured value)	Variable data (continuous value)
p Chart	Attribute data (discrete value)
np Chart	Attribute data (discrete value)
c Chart	Attribute data (discrete value)
u Chart	Attribute data (discrete value)

Table 4-13. Description of the various types of control charts.

Chart Type	Chart Description
X̄ (X-bar) R Chart	This is a two-part chart used for monitoring processes that generate continuous data. The X-bar chart monitors the accuracy of a process, while the R monitors the precision of a process. The absence of accuracy is reflected in the excessive variability between samples, and the absence of precision is reflected in the excessive variability within samples. It is used for data such as patient waiting time and food temperature.
p Chart	The p chart is used to chart the results of a process which generates attribute data. It is applied to problems pertaining to the percentage of a service which are unacceptable/acceptable, such as percentage medication errors, percentage patient billing error, and percentage of patients readmitted for the same problem within a specified time period.
np Chart	This is a special type of the p chart, where instead of the percentage of non-conformance, the number of non-conforming service is tracked, e.g., the number of medication errors found in lots of equal sample size.
c Chart	This chart is used for attribute data. It is an area-of-opportunity chart with equal areas. An example is the number of accidents reported per day. The opportunity for the occurrence of the event must be constant.
u Chart	u charts serve the same basic purpose as the c charts; however, the opportunity for occurrence of the event is not the same. An example is the number of misdiagnoses per DRG.

Procedure for Constructing a p Chart

Step 1. Plot the fraction of billing errors against time. Select an appropriate scale for both axes. The y-axis is the *percentage billing error* and the x-axis is the *day*. See Figure 4-25. Use dots to indicate each pair of data.

Step 2. Connect the points with straight lines consecutively.

Step 3. Establish the control limits using the equations presented below:

The centerline for a p chart is also the average of the samples taken.

Table 4-14. Billing error information.

Day	Number of Records Inspected	Number of Billing Errors	Fraction of Billing Errors
1	100	2	.020
2	100	0	.000
3	100	5	.050
4	100	5	.050
5	100	3	.030
6	100	2	.020
7	100	4	.040
8	100	5	.050
9	100	2	.020
10	100	3	.030
11	100	1	.010
12	100	4	.040
13	100	2	.020
14	100	0	.000
15	100	3	.030
16	100	1	.010
17	100	2	.020
18	100	1	.010
19	100	10	.100
20	100	9	.090
21	100	3	.030
22	100	2	.020
23	100	3	.030
24	100	0	.000
25	100	3	.030
	2500	75	

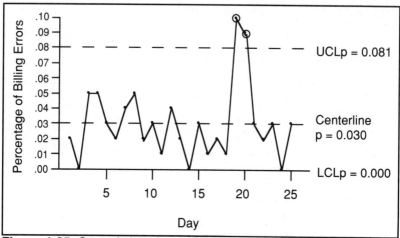

Figure 4-25. Control chart for percentage billing error.

$$p = \frac{\text{Total number of billing errors examined}}{\text{Total number of units examined}}$$

p = 75/2500 = 0.030

   The control limits are set at the value of p plus and minus three times the standard error.

Upper Control Limit (UCLp) $= p + 3\sqrt{[p(1-p)/n]}$

Lower Control Limit (LCLp) $= p - 3\sqrt{[p(1-p)/n]}$

where
n is the size of the subgroup = 100

Calculations:

i) Centerline = p = 0.030

ii) UCLp $= 0.030 + 3\sqrt{[0.03(0.97)/100]}$
$$= 0.030 + 0.051$$
$$= 0.081$$

Therefore, the upper control limit = 0.081

iii) $LCLp = 0.030 - 3\sqrt{[0.03(0.97)/100]}$

   $= 0.030 - 0.051$

   $= -0.021$

Note: Since a negative percentage billing error is not possible, the lower control limit is set at 0.000.

Therefore, the lower control limit = 0.00

How to Use Control Charts to Stabilize a Process

Once the control chart has been plotted, the next step is to detect the presence of any variations due to special causes. The process showed in Figure 4-25 is said to be "out-of-control" since not all of the plotted points are within the control limits. The control chart seems to show that on days 19 and 20, something unusually bad occurred. It is also worth noting that that the occurrences on days 2 and 24 are within the system, thus showing that the system is capable of zero billing errors (2 out of 25 days).

For days 19 and 20, it can be inferred that a special variation occurred. Once a hospital manager determines that the cause of a variation is special, he or she must take steps toward eliminating it permanently. Policies must be put into effect to prevent a recurrence.

The information obtained for days 2 and 24 indicate that the process is truly capable of producing zero billing errors. These should not be treated like special cause days.

Bringing the Process Under Control

Suppose that management investigated the points that were out-of-control (days 19 and 20) so as to identify and eliminate the special cause of variation in the process. During the investigation, the hospital management found that on days 19 and 20 a newly hired billing clerk was put in charge of patient billing without any training. It is then concluded that this change in the work structure could have been responsible for the variation. To permanently correct this problem the hospital instituted a one-day in-house training program for all new billing clerks.

After taking appropriate action to prevent a recurrence of the special causes, the data from days 19 and 20 are deleted and a new control chart was constructed as shown in Figure 4-26.

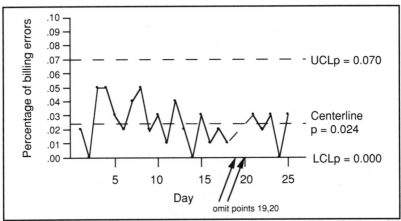

Figure 4-26. Control chart of the process after eliminating the special causes of variation.

Recalculation of Control Limits

$$p = \text{Centerline} = (75 - 19) / 2300 = 56 / 2300 = 0.024$$

$$UCLp = 0.024 + 3\sqrt{[0.024(1 - 0.024)/100]}$$
$$= 0.024 + 3(0.0153)$$
$$= 0.0699 \approx 0.070$$

$$LCLp = 0.024 - 3(0.0153)$$
$$= -0.022$$
$$= 0.000$$

Note that the out-of-control points have been removed. The newly drawn control chart may still have other out-of-control points due to narrower limits. Such points should also be investigated for special causes. Several such iterations may be needed to stabilize the process and bring it under control.

Table 4-15. Control chart formulas.

Type of Chart	Formula	Explanations / Comments
$\overline{X}$ Chart	$UCL = \overline{\overline{X}} + A_2R$ $Centerline = \overline{\overline{X}}$ $LCL = \overline{\overline{X}} - A_2R$	Monitors the accuracy of a process $\overline{X}$ = Average value of each subgroup $\overline{\overline{X}}$ = Sum of $\overline{X}$ divided by the number of subgroups. See Table 4-16 for the A_2 values.
R Chart	$UCL = D_4\overline{R}$ $Centerline = \overline{R}$ $LCL = D_3\overline{R}$	Monitors the precision of a process R = Range = difference between the minimum and the maximum values of the data in a subgroup. $\overline{R}$ = the average of all range values for each subgroup. The D_3 and D_4 values can be found in Table 4-16.
np Chart	$UCL =$ $np + 3\sqrt{np\,(1 - np)}$ $Centerline = np$ $LCL =$ $np - 3\sqrt{np\,(1 - np)}$	Used for sample of constant size. Same as a p chart, except that the number of unacceptable unit of service is used rather than the fraction unacceptable.
c Chart	$UCL = \overline{c} + 3\sqrt{\overline{c}}$ $Centerline = \overline{c}$ $LCL = \overline{c} - 3\sqrt{\overline{c}}$	The conditions that generate each subgroup must be the same. Health care applications are not very common.
u Chart	$UCL = \overline{u} + 3\sqrt{\overline{u} - n}$ $Centerline = \overline{u}$ $LCL = \overline{u} - 3\sqrt{\overline{u} - n}$	The conditions that generate each subgroup could vary. Health care applications are not very common.

QUALITY OF CARE (QC) STORY

The preceding portions of this chapter have demonstrated how quality control tools can be used in identifying problems and solutions pertaining to customers. The QC Story (Figure 4-27) is a logical format for presenting the history of the improvement

Table 4-16. Control chart constants.

Number of Observations in Subgroup, n	A₂	A₃	B₃	B₄	C₄	d₂	d₃	D₃	D₄	E₂
2	1.880	2.659	0.000	3.267	0.7979	1.128	0.853	0.000	3.267	2.660
3	1.023	1.954	0.000	2.568	0.8862	1.693	0.888	0.000	2.574	1.772
4	0.729	1.628	0.000	2.266	0.9213	2.059	0.880	0.000	2.282	1.457
5	0.577	1.427	0.000	2.089	0.9400	2.326	0.864	0.000	2.114	1.290
6	0.483	1.287	0.030	1.970	0.9515	2.534	0.848	0.000	2.004	1.184
7	0.419	1.182	0.118	1.882	0.9594	2.704	0.833	0.076	1.924	1.109
8	0.373	1.099	0.185	1.815	0.9650	2.847	0.820	0.136	1.864	1.054
9	0.337	1.032	0.239	1.761	0.9693	2.970	0.808	0.184	1.816	1.010
10	0.308	0.975	0.284	1.716	0.9727	3.078	0.797	0.223	1.777	0.975
11	0.285	0.927	0.321	1.679	0.9754	3.173	0.787	0.256	1.744	
12	0.266	0.886	0.354	1.646	0.9776	3.258	0.778	0.283	1.717	
13	0.249	0.850	0.382	1.618	0.9794	3.336	0.770	0.307	1.693	
14	0.235	0.817	0.406	1.594	0.9810	3.407	0.762	0.328	1.672	
15	0.223	0.789	0.428	1.572	0.9823	3.472	0.755	0.347	1.653	
16	0.212	0.763	0.448	1.552	0.9835	3.532	0.749	0.363	1.637	
17	0.203	0.739	0.466	1.534	0.9845	3.588	0.743	0.378	1.622	
18	0.194	0.718	0.482	1.518	0.9854	3.640	0.738	0.391	1.608	
19	0.187	0.698	0.497	1.503	0.9862	3.689	0.733	0.403	1.597	
20	0.180	0.680	0.510	1.490	0.9869	3.735	0.729	0.415	1.585	
21	0.173	0.663	0.523	1.477	0.9876	3.778	0.724	0.425	1.575	
22	0.167	0.647	0.534	1.466	0.9882	3.819	0.720	0.434	1.566	
23	0.162	0.633	0.545	1.455	0.9887	3.858	0.716	0.443	1.557	
24	0.157	0.619	0.555	1.445	0.9892	3.895	0.712	0.451	1.548	
25	0.153	0.606	0.565	1.435	0.9896	3.931	0.709	0.459	1.541	
More than 25	$3/\sqrt{n}$		$1-3/\sqrt{2n}$	$1+3/\sqrt{2n}$						

Copyright ASTM. Reprinted with permission, from ASTM Manual on the Presentation of Data and Control Chart Analysis (1976, pgs. 134-136).

QUALITY OF CARE (QC) STORY

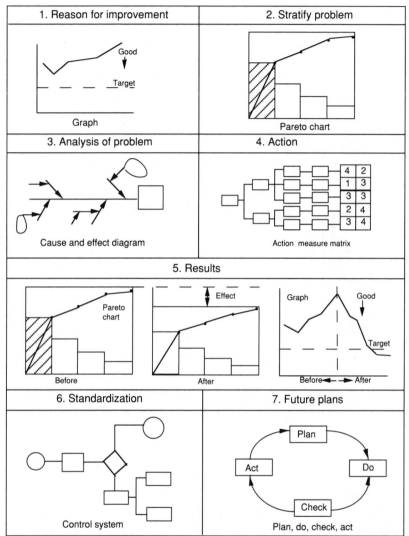

Figure 4-27. The QC Story.

process—identification of the improvement opportunity area, analysis of the problem, and solution of the problem. The QC Story helps teams to organize, gather, and analyze information, and monitor the team's progress. It is used to illustrate and communicate the team's problem-solving process. Its presentation makes it possible for non-team members to understand the improvement process. It also makes it easy to solicit input from non-team members. Figure 4-28 is an example of the action matrix.

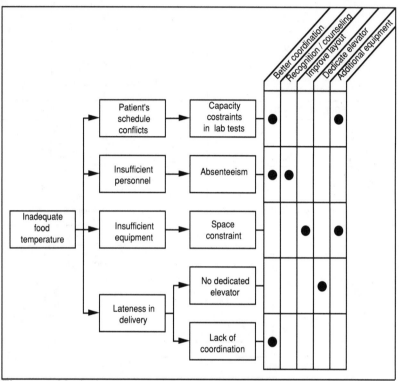

Figure 4-28. Action measures matrix for the food temperature problem.

The QC Story serves as a guide for PDCA. If presented correctly, it will provide both the team, and others, with a complete picture of the logical process used for improvement. The QC Story is used at every stage of the team's activities and every step of the improvement process. The following steps are required in order to develop a QC Story:

Step 1. Determine the reason for improvement:
• What needs to be controlled?
• What makes improvement imperative?
• What are the consequences of improving or not improving?
• How does the problem affect the customer?

Step 2. *Stratify the general into its component parts:*
• Divide the problem into parts.
• Look at the problem in many different ways.
• Look for areas of significance and impact.
• Choose the area of greatest significance under the team's control.
• Set a target for improvement.

Step 3. *Analysis of the problem:*
• Determine why the problem exists.
• Verify cause(s) with data.
• Quantify their effect on the problem.

Step 4. *Action-measures:*
• Propose methods to eliminate the cause(s) of the problem.
• Select the best solution on the basis of feasibility, effectiveness, and impact.
• Plan how to implement the solution (action-measures).

Step 5. *Results:*
• Check to determine if the action-measures taken are successful in eliminating the causes of the problem.
• Did the overall performance indicator improve to the targeted level set in step 2?
• If not, return to steps 3 and 4 to take further corrective action.

Step 6. *Standardization and formalization:*
• Maintain the gains achieved.
• Build (or implement) the improvement into the normal course of business to ensure continued results.

Step 7. *Future plans:*
• Would additional (more important) benefits be achieved if another part of the problem was solved?
• What lessons have been learned by the team that will help in solving their next problem?

QUALITY FUNCTION DEPLOYMENT

Quality Function Deployment (QFD) is a system for designing product or service based on customer demands and involving all members of the producer or supplier organization. It is sometimes referred to as the most advanced form of Total Quality Control, Japanese style. The following case study illustrates how QFD would work in a health-care environment.

A Case Example

Suppose that a hospital (through customer surveys) compiled a list of customer demands as shown in Figure 4-29. The demands should be stated in positive terms. For example, a patient's complaint over the noise level in the nursing unit can be translated into a positive demand by stating it as a desire for a *quiet atmosphere*. Similarly, complaints of rudeness of staff and failure to respond promptly to call lights can be restated in terms of the

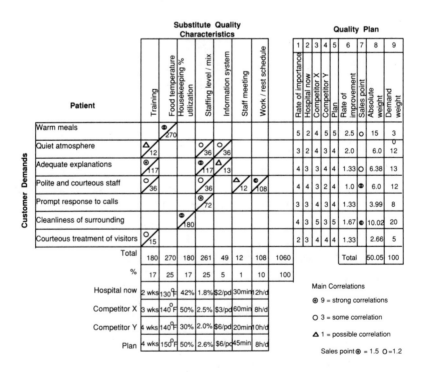

Figure 4-29. Applying QFD to a hospital.

customer's desire for a *polite and courteous staff,* and *prompt response to call lights.* A QFD chart to assist the hospital in better designing the services it provides so as to meet the needs of the patients.

The customer demands used in this example are selected for simplicity. It is also possible to perform this exercise using customer demands such as "make me better," "receive accurate diagnosis," and "receive correct medication." Many customer demands come in the form of language data, which may not be easily translated into quantifiable information. Language data must be properly compiled and managed. It should not be treated as throw-away information.

How to Complete a QFD Chart

Column 1: The *rate of importance* is a rating of the customer demands on a scale of 1 to 5, with 5 being most important and 1 being of relatively low importance. These ratings should be done by the customers (patients or any of the other customer groups in health care, such as physicians, insurance, patient families, etc.). It is better to use the demands from one class of customers at a time. Customer surveys represent the best source of this information. There are also publications that compare hospitals on the basis of some customer related criteria. Such publications would also be an adequate source of rating information.

In our example, *warm meals* was ranked highest, while *adequate explanations, polite and courteous staff,* and *cleanliness of surroundings* were ranked next highest.

Column 2: *Hospital now* lists where the hospital is today on each of the customer demands listed, on a scale of 1 to 5, with 5 being very good and 1 being very poor. Again, rating information should be provided by the customers through patient (customer) surveys.

Columns 3 and 4: *Competitor X and competitor Y* provides a listing of how two of your primary competitors are doing with respect to each customer demand on a scale of 1 to 5. A good customer survey conducted by an outside independent agency can be used to successfully gather information regarding you and your competitors. Also, some trade magazines do comparative reporting. More competitors may be looked at if data about them can be obtained or if they are industry leaders.

Column 5: *Plan* is an indication of where the hospital is heading with respect to each of the customer demands. This is determined by looking at where the hospital is today, *hospital now*, and what the competitors are doing with respect to the customer demands. It also takes into account the hospital's strategic plan and policy deployment.

Column 6: *Rate of improvement* is determined by dividing where the hospital plans to be, column 5 by where the hospital is today, column 2.

Column 7: *Sales point* indicates which patient (customer) demands are the most important marketing theme for the hospital. A double circle or 1.5 is used to indicate a strong sales point; a circle or 1.2 is used for a lesser sales point; and a blank or 1.0 is used for items which are not sales points. It is impractical to make every customer demand a sales point.

Column 8: *Absolute (quality) weight* is determined by multiplying the rate of importance (column 1) by the rate of improvement (column 6) and multiplying the result by the sales point (column 7).

$$\text{Absolute weight} = \text{col. 1} \times \text{col. 6} \times \text{col. 7}$$

Column 9: *Demand (quality) weight* is determined by converting the absolute (quality) weight to a percentage, i.e., divide the total of column 8 into each item to get the percentage of each item.

The purpose of this part of the exercise is then achieved by identifying the most important customer demands to work on. In our case, the top customer demands are warm meals, with a weight of 30 percent; cleanliness of surrounding, with a weight of 20 percent; and adequate explanations, with a weight of 13 percent.

Substitute Quality Characteristics

Substitute quality characteristics are the items that are controlled by the organization; they may or may not satisfy customer demands. When for example, patients express the need for *good meals,* one of the ways in which a health-care organization can control that specific demand is by translating it into the *nutritional content (value)* of the meals served. This is one of the important functions of QFD. Substitute quality characteristics are generated for each of the customer demands. Substitute quality characteristics can be gathered through brainstorming and subsequent grouping of related items. Each substitute quality characteristic represents a controllable response which must be examined to see if implementing it will meet the needs of the individual customer demands. The quality characteristics and their specific controllable variables are presented below.

- *Training:* length of training in weeks.

- *Food temperature:* food temperature measured in degree Fahrenheit.
- *Housekeeping percent utilization:* measured as a ratio of housekeeping actual hours to available hours.

- *Staffing level and mix:* measured as the combined daily unit ratio of the number of RNs to the number of patients multiplied by the number of nurses to the number of patients:

$$\frac{\text{number of RNs}}{\text{number of patients}} \times \frac{\text{number of nurses}}{\text{number of patients}}$$

The combined number of nurses will include all the nurses in the unit—RNs, LPNs, and NAs. For example, if a nursing unit with 30 patients is staffed with 2 RNs, 4 LPNs, and 2 NAs, then the staffing level and mix indicator will be given as

$$(2/30) \times (8/30) = 0.0178 = 1.8\%$$

Notice that the combined ratio by itself is not sufficient because even if there are 20 nurses to 30 patients, it may take an RN to adequately explain a medication or procedure to the patient. On the other hand, when it comes to answering call lights promptly, it may essentially require that the overall ratio of combined nursing staff to patients be high, irrespective of the mix.

- *Information system:* information system, such as a noisy printer, may be partly responsible for noise in the nursing unit. Also, if the information is complete and promptly available via some department-to-unit transfer (such as test results), the nurses might be able to provide adequate explanations to patients. Hence the best indicator of the adequacy of the information system is the average amount spent on information systems per patient day. This is estimated for this hospital as $2 per patient day. By slightly increasing this amount, the hospital units may be able to eliminate the noise and have a faster means of transmitting information to the units.

- *Staff meetings:* staff meetings are important for staff development, among other reasons. The only constraint has to be in the amount of time spent on meetings per week. If meeting time can be increased from 30 minutes per week to 45 minutes per week, each unit might have enough time to cover normal operating issues as well as to instruct its staff on the importance of politeness and courtesy towards patients.

- *Work and rest schedule:* perhaps the most often cited reason for rudeness of staff is due to tiredness and fatigue from excessively long number of working hours in one stretch. When nurses work for 12 hours or more per day, they tend to become irritable and sometimes rude, especially during the last couple of hours. The hospital's plan could be to reduce the number of hours per day from 12 to 10.

Each organization is different and may have other more appropriate ways of arriving at a measurable indicator for the substitute quality characteristics.

Correlations

Once the substitute characteristics have been broken down to a measurable level, the next step is to determine if and when there is a correlation between the customer demands and the quality characteristics. A double circle (9 points) is used to denote strong correlation (as in *warm meals* and *food temperature*), a single circle (3 points) denotes some correlation, and a triangle (1 point) denotes possible correlation. The number beneath each symbol entry is arrived at by multiplying the demand weight by the equivalent symbol points. As an example, the correlation symbol between warm meals and food temperature is equivalent to 9 points, and the corresponding demand weight is 30. Hence the entry below the diagonal is given as 9 x 30 = 270.

Interpreting Bottom Rows

- The *total* row is the summation of the numerical values beneath the symbols. For example, the total number of points for *training* is 12 + 117 + 36 + 15 = 180.

- *Percentage (%)* is an expression of each subtotal as a percentage of the grand total. For example, for *staffing level* and *mix*, it is given as 261 / 1060 x 100 = 25%
- *Hospital now* is a quantifiable indicator representing where the hospital is today with respect to each substitute characteristic. The values in this row must be measurable. The following is an explanation of how each measurable criterion was derived:

  —*Training:* The hospital presently provides 2 weeks of training to its new nursing employees. It plans to do better than this figure in the future.

  —*Food temperature:* The average food temperature today is about 130°F. There is a need to improve upon this figure.

  —*Housekeeping utilization percentage:* Presently, the housekeeping department works for 10 hours out of a possible 24 hours in a day. This gives it a utilization factor of 10 / 24 x 100 = 42%. If cleanliness is a concern of the patients, then, the hospital may wish to increase the utilization factor.

—*Staffing level and mix:* As explained earlier under substitute characteristics, staffing level and mix can be assessed by using the formula below:

$$\frac{\text{number of RNs}}{\text{unit census}} \times \frac{\text{combined number of nurses}}{\text{unit census}} \times 100$$

While this index by itself may offer no meaning, its change from one period to another will affect some of the customer demands such as *adequate explanations* and *prompt response to call lights.* Also, a plain ratio of nurses to patients may be suitable in certain situations. For this hospital's unit, this indicator is 1.8 percent.

—*Information systems:* This value is stated in terms of dollars per patient day. Presently, this value is $2 per patient day.

—*Staff meeting:* Presently, the nursing unit spends 30 minutes per week for staff meetings. It may wish to increase this time in order to formally present more facts on the impact of staff behavior on patients.
—*Work/rest schedule:* The manner in which work and rest is scheduled has often been linked to stress and fatigue in staff members. Presently, nursing staff members work 12-hour shifts. The hospital may wish to reduce this number.

- *Competitors X and Y:* represent how the primary competing hospitals are performing with respect to the substitute quality characteristics discussed above.

- *Plan:* represents where the hospital plans to be in the future. This is a list of the target values for each substitute quality characteristic based on a review of each competitor.

Conclusions

The following conclusions can be drawn from this exercise:

• The two most important patient demands are *warm meals* and *cleanliness of surrounding*, each with a demand weight of 30 and 20 respectively.

• The two most important substitute quality characteristics are *food temperature* and *staffing level and mix*, each with a total of 270 and 261 points respectively. *Housekeeping* and *training* are also calling for a high priority status.

• Once target values have been set, the next step is to utilize strategic planning and policy deployment to determine how these planned targets will be achieved. Once achieved, the gains must be preserved through the practice of quality in daily work.

ROAD MAP FOR THE IMPLEMENTATION OF TQM

Transforming a hospital organization by inspiring its administrators, clinical and non-clinical staff to embrace the philosophy of never-ending improvement requires conviction, hard work, determination, and constant affirmation and reaffirmation at the highest levels. This process cannot take place overnight. It is not sufficient for the transformation to occur at a departmental level or among individuals. It has to be organization-wide. The commitment of top management must be unequivocal. Anything less is a recipe for failure. Management and employees must be enthusiastic about and committed to the idea of learning from all types of customers (patients, physicians, third party payers, internal customers, the community, etc), what their expectations are.

It is possible for a hospital to fail financially and close its doors even when every department is doing its job efficiently. As a result of the level of competition in health care today, simply maintaining an existing quality level, even a good one, is not sufficient. One of the major challenges facing health-care organizations today is that of mastering the art and science of continuous quality improvement, and making it a permanent component of its total business philosophy. Total Quality Management must be approached as an integrated activity with the customers being the ultimate beneficiary. Improvement should not be a specific (or static) goal. It should be a moving target; one that is continually reset at higher levels as the old levels are reached.

Figure 4-30 presents a road map for the implementation of TQM in healthcare organizations. The mission statement of an organization must reflect the purpose of the organization, its long term objectives towards its customers and its employees. Once developed, policy management should be employed to make it possible for everyone in the organization to become familiar with the mission statement. In addition, management must also commit to educating the employees and preparing them for the cultural change. The transformation cannot be immediate. It must be deliberate and gradual.

One way to facilitate the process of transformation is to identify key individuals within the health-care organization who already have a disposition towards change. Test cases can then be implemented within the departments of such individuals. It is important to vigorously publicize the activities of test groups or teams, as well as their results. Management should not intimidate employees into team membership or any form of participation. It is however within the purview of a commited management philosophy to provide the right incentives and work environment to encourage voluntary participation in QC Circles. A necessary starting point lies in the adaptation of Dr. Deming's 14 points.

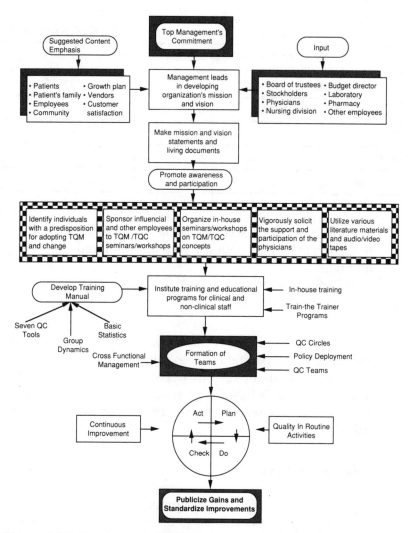

Figure 4-30. Road map to TQM implementation in health-care organizations.

EXERCISES

4-1. The XYZ hospital is interested in applying the concept of TQC in reducing the number of patients delivering by Caesarean section (C-section) so as to decrease patient risk and increase patient satisfaction. A study of the problem revealed the following causes of the problem.

Cause	Percent Occurrence
1. Cephalo-pelvic disproportion (a problem with the ratio of the infant's head to the mother's pelvis) or failure to progress.	40 %
2. Infants in breech position	16 %
3. Fetal distress	14%
4. Previous births by C-section	13%
5. All other causes	17%

a) Perform a Pareto analysis using the given data.
b) Generate similar data for your hospital and do the following:
   i) Pareto analysis
   ii) Cause and effect diagram

4-2. Suppose that the biomedical (clinical) engineering department of a local hospital receives calls for equipment service from individuals in various departments of the hospital. The data below is based on a study of 107 source requests to determine the reasons for the calls and the frequency of calls.

Reasons for the Call   **Frequency**

1. Staff forgot how to use equipment   25
2. Staff not properly trained to use equipment   42
3. Equipment breakdown (down)   18
4. Equipment malfunction   10
5. Other   12

a) Perform a Pareto analysis of the problem.
b) Perform an actual analysis of the problem at your facility.
c) What factors are commonly responsible for the inadequate training of the staff? What training methods are being used and how effective are they?

4-3. The data below shows the waiting times (in minutes) for patients in queue for a CT SCAN at a local hospital.

a)Perform a histogram on the data. What deductions can you make from the histogram?

Waiting Times for CT SCAN (min.)

10	15	2	40	35	22
62	40	47	22	33	52
11	17	28	18	39	43
31	39	36	12	42	15
43	19	11	62	65	40
13	18	14	20	21	8

b) Suppose that a study revealed the causes of delays to be as follows:

• Failure of technician to correctly indicate what needs to be done
• Patient not scheduled in advance
• Doctor not available
• Patient arrives late
• Technician not aware that patient is waiting
• Delays in verifying patient's insurance

Draw a cause and effect diagram to reflect the causes of such delays (if they exist) at your facility. Use a pie chart to show the breakdown of causes.

c) Perform a similar analysis for ultrasound, nuclear medicine, and X-rays.

4-4. Answer the following questions and apply two or more of the TQC tools presented in the chapter to analyze the information gathered in each question. What are the implications for quality improvement ?

a) How do the mortality and morbidity rates in your hospital compare (on a severity adjusted basis) to the regional and national standards? Use at least five years of data if available.

b) Study the average elapsed time from the initiation of a radiology order by a physician to the time that the results become available.

c) Determine the average number of complaints from patients due to incorrect billing during the past six months?

BIBLIOGRAPHY

Batchelor, G. J. and R. Graham. 1989. Quality management in nursing. *Journal of Society of Health Systems*. 1:63-68.

Berwick, D. M. Continuous improvement as an ideal in health care. *New England Journal of Medicine*. 320:53-56.

Bradford, R. 1989. Obstacles to collaborative practice. *Nursing Management*. 20(4):72.

Crosby, P. B. 1984. *Quality Without Tears: The Art of Hassle-free Management*. New York: McGraw-Hill Book Company.

_____. *Quality is Free: The Art of Making Quality Certain*. New York: McGraw-Hill Book Company.

Darr, K. 1989. Applying the Deming method in hospitals: Part 2. *Hospital Topics*. 68(1):4.

Dasbach, E. J. and D. Gustafson. 1989. Impacting quality in health care: The role of the health systems engineer. *Journal of the Society for Health Systems*. 1(1):75-84.

Deming, W. E. 1986. *Out of the Crises*. Cambridge, MA: Massachusetts Institute of Technology.

_____. 1986. Drastic changes for western management. Gold Coast City, Australia. Paper presented at the The Institute of Management Sciences meeting.

Demos, M. P. and N. Demos. 1989. Statistical quality control's role in health care management. *Quality Progress*. August.

Donabedian, A. 1978. The quality of medical care. *Science*. 200:856-864.

Feigenbaum, A. V. 1983. *Total Quality Control*. New York: McGraw Hill Book Company.

Garvin, D. A. 1988. *Managing Quality: The Strategic and Competitive Edge*. New York: The Free Press.

Gitlow, H., S. Gitlow, A. Oppenheim, and R. Oppenheim. 1989. *Tools and Methods for Improvement of Quality*. Homewood, IL: Irwin Publishers.

Goldberg, A. M. 1984. *Quality Circles in Health Care Facilities: A Model for Excellence*. Rockville, MD: Aspen Systems Corporation.

Hart, M. K. and R. Hart. 1989. *Quantitative Methods for Quality and Productivity Improvement*. Milwaukee, WI: Quality Press.

Hauser, J. R. and D. Clausing. 1988. The house of quality. *Harvard Business Review*. May-June. p. 63-73.

Hayes, G. E. 1985. *Quality and Productivity: The New Challenge*. Wheaton, IL: Hitchcock Executive Book Science.

Ishikawa, K. 1985. *What Is Total Quality Control?* Translated by David J. Lu. Englewood Cliffs, NJ: Prentice-Hall.

_____. 1982. *Guide to Quality Control*. Tokyo, Japan: Asian Productivity Organization, Kraus International Publications.

Juran, J. M. 1988. *Juran on Planning for Quality.* New York: The Free Press.

_____. 1986. The quality trilogy. *Quality Progress.* 19(8):19-24.

Kano, N. 1988. Administrative systems for TQC. Lecture Series, University of Miami.

King, B. 1987. *Better Design in Half the Time.* Massachusetts: GOAL/QPC.

Kume, Hitoshi. 1985. *Statistical Methods for Quality Improvement.* Tokyo, Japan: AOTS Chosakai, Ltd.

Mann, N. R. 1989. *The Keys to Excellence.* Los Angeles, CA: Prestwick Books.

Micheletti, J. A. and T. Shlala. 1989. Quality assurance in ancillary departments. *Journal of the Society for Health Systems.* 1(1):69-73.

Milakovich, M. 1989. Working paper: Implementing total health care quality improvement: A conceptual guide for health care administrators and managers. Coral Gables, FL: University of Miami.

Montgomery, D. C. 1985. *Introduction to Statistical Quality Control.* New York: John Wiley & Sons, Inc.

Nackel, J. G. and T. Collier. 1989. Implementing a quality improvement program. *Journal of the Society for Health Systems.* 1(1):85-100.

Omachonu, V. K. 1989. Quality of care and the patient: New criteria for evaluation. *Health Care Management Review.* 15(4).

Omachonu, V. K. and M. Beruvides. 1989. Improving hospital productivity: Patient-, unit-, and hospital-based measures. *Proceedings of IIE International Industrial Engineering Conference.* Norcross, GA: Institute of Industrial Engineers.

Rosander, A. C. 1989. *The Quest for Quality on Services*. Milwaukee, WI: Quality Press and White Plains, NY: Quality Resources.

Sahney, V. K., J. I. Dutkewych, and W. R. Schramm. 1989. Quality improvement process: The foundation for excellence in health care. *Journal of the Society for Health Systems*. 1(1):17-29.

Scherkenbach, W. *The Deming Route to Quality and Productivity*. Milwaukee, WI: Quality Press.

Ullmann, S. G. 1985. The impact of quality on cost in the provision of long-term care. *Inquiry*. 22:293-302.

Walsh, L., R. Wurster, and R. Kimbler (eds.). 1986. *Quality Management Handbook*. New York: Marcel Dekker and Milwaukee, WI: Quality Press.

Part Three

Productivity and Cost Containment in Health Care

This section discusses the concepts of productivity, profitability, price recovery, and efficiency in health-care organizations. It explains the various components of the cost of resources consumed in the delivery of health care.

Chapter Five discusses the limitations of present definitions of productivity, presents practical approaches for measuring the total productivity of a nursing unit, and discusses diagnoses-based productivity.

Chapter Six explores the relationship between the components of productivity, profitability, and price-recovery. The application of the Multi Factor Productivity Measurement Model (MFPMM) is also presented.

In Chapter Seven, various productivity improvement strategies are presented, followed by a discussion on how each strategy would affect the productivity equation. Attempts are made to clearly show how each strategy would lead to productivity increases.

Chapter Eight examines the role of physicians in the creation and control of costs. The link is made between physicians' characteristics and practice patterns, as well as between physicians' characteristics and costs. The chapter concludes with a discussion on how to monitor physicians' practice patterns to achieve cost containment.

5 Productivity Measurement

The measurement of productivity in health care is a subject that has generated wide interest among researchers and practitioners. Difficulties in developing acceptable measurement models have given rise to the use of various types of performance indicators in place of formal productivity measures. Productivity is a subset of quality; gains in productivity should not be pursued independent of improvement in quality. Increased productivity is a direct result of improved quality. A comprehensive productivity measurement model should reflect the following key components:

- the total resources consumed (not just one or some) in the delivery of health care

- the context in which nursing and medical care occur, such as a nursing unit or an outpatient unit

- built-in implications for productivity improvement through changes in levels of output and input

- the link between productivity and quality of care

- input and output values in constant dollars and the built-in implications for profitability

Although doctors are primarily responsible for the generation and control of costs, nurses are in the best position to monitor and manage resource consumption at the point of consumption. Therefore, this chapter focuses on costs generated in the nursing unit.

Productivity measurement should begin with a complete definition of productivity. Some of the definitions being used today are incomplete, for example:

- Productivity measures which define output as the quantity of service rendered (stated as number of nursing hours available) per unit of time, leave much to be desired. Such measures ignore the traditional concepts of productivity which define output in terms of value of services rendered. Also, the process of caring for patients is very complex and is made up of tangible and intangible components; it is difficult to determine what, therefore, constitutes the "quantity" of health care services. Another difficulty with this definition is that it is not easily distinguishable from the input of the system, which also includes nursing care hours.

- Some definitions of productivity compare actual nursing care hours to required nursing care hours. These are definitions of efficiency rather than productivity. Efficiency is defined as the ratio of actual output attained to standard output expected. Also, such a definition implies that productivity can be increased by reducing the required nursing care hours or by increasing the number of actual nursing care hours. A valid productivity measurement model must present a clear understanding of prospects for productivity improvement.

- Perhaps the most common definition of nursing productivity is the one stated as "hours per patient day." Such a definition considers only the cost of direct nursing care and ignores indirect nursing care, ancillary, and overhead costs. A clear distinction should be made between a performance indicator designed for the purpose of monitoring one parameter of a system and a formal and dynamic program of productivity management based on total resources consumed.

In addition to a valid outcome-based measure, a definition of productivity including the context in which care is provided is needed. Today's productivity measurement models should be driven by DRGs (or other forms of diagnosis classification system in use) and should consider the effect of all resources consumed in the delivery of care, not just direct labor resources. Such measures should be simple, quantifiable, and able to undergo cost analysis. Such a vast network of complex interrelationships exists among input resources, processes, and outputs that it will be difficult to find one category of measurement or one definition that captures the whole essence of productivity. Of immense necessity, therefore, is an operational framework showing the interrelationship among the several (quantifiable) factors affecting productivity.

It should be stated that a productivity measure by itself is of no use except when compared with a similar measure during another time period, or when used for planning and assessment purposes.

OUTCOME-BASED AND OUTPUT-BASED MEASURES

Two broad concepts of nursing productivity have been proposed in health-care literature: *outcome* and *output* productivity. *Outcome* measures consider the results of nursing intervention, such as the ability to restore good health to a patient, or to enhance a peaceful death. *Output* measures, on the other hand, focus on the dollar value of the services rendered and resources expended.

For a long time, developing *outcome*-based measures has confounded those in nursing and associated disciplines owing to the complex and subjective nature of their intervening variables. Figure 5-1 shows a conceptual framework for an *outcome*-based productivity measurement model. It is generally agreed that more work is needed on the subject of outcome measures.

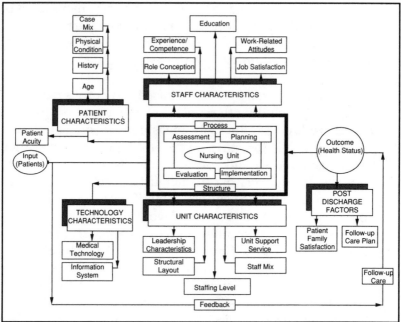

Figure 5-1. A conceptual framework for an outcome-based productivity measure.

Measuring productivity using *output-based* measures has become necessary only recently. Prior to DRGs, there was virtually no incentive to the hospital for cost containment. The mandate to base health-care payments on prospective pricing now forces hospitals to recognize the importance of *output* measures.

With DRGs in effect, the products of hospitals are now somewhat definable. As a result, the following research opportunities have emerged:

• Researching questions regarding profitability, productivity, and quality of care which have resulted from gathering closely related DRGs to form various product lines.

• Studying output measures to understand and contain health-care costs.

The concept of DRGs has heightened interest in product line definition and management. Although far from perfect, DRGs have established a consistent measure which facilitates comparisons across all hospitals.

Output-Based Productivity Measures

In hospitals, care delivery occurs around the clock and involves a wide range of complex activities, including management, coordination, education, and direct patient care. The nursing unit is the point of focus for direct patient care and is ultimately the front line of hospital operations. A nursing unit is analogous to an operational unit such as a factory floor where resources go through a process of transformation to produce finished goods (see figure 5-2). By looking at a nursing unit in this way, resource consumption and quality of care can be observed and monitored. All resources consumed in the process can be evaluated instead of only direct nursing care hours. Ancillary services make up a major part of the product but are often ignored by many measures. Nursing unit productivity measures can be used among competing units within a hospital as well as between similar units of different hospitals.

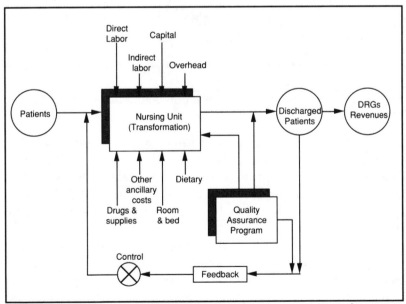

Figure 5-2. Schematic of nursing unit patient care resource inputs and outputs.

A conceptual framework showing the relationships among the different variables of inputs and outputs is essential in the development of a productivity measurement model. Such a conceptual framework is shown in Figure 5-3. One of the important features of this conceptual framework is its ability to examine care delivery in an institutional context.

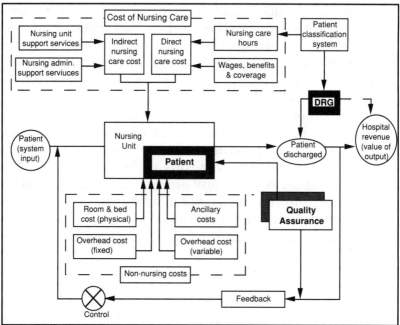

Figure 5-3. Conceptual framework for an output-based productivity measure.

Quality assurance is a very important component of this output-based conceptual framework. The ongoing unit-related quality assurance program of a given hospital can be integrated into it, although the ideal situation calls for a TQM-driven quality assurance program of which productivity management is a part.

Once a patient departs the system (hospital unit), healthcare management is expected to draw upon the experiences of treating that patient for future use. Similarly, productivity measurement, improvement, cost reduction, and quality assurance should be a dynamic and ever-present component of the process as depicted by the feedback loop.

Determining Inputs for Productivity Measurement

Resource inputs for the patient treatment at a hospital can be divided into nursing care costs and non-nursing care costs. Physician costs are not included since they have the opportunity of billing separately. Nursing care costs are further broken down into direct and indirect nursing care costs.

Direct nursing care costs are those costs associated with the nursing care hours of registered nurses (RNs), licensed practical nurses (LPNs), and nurse's aides (NAs). Indirect nursing care costs are those associated with the hours spent by the nursing unit support services and nursing administration support services. Nursing unit support services are made up of the head nurse, the charge nurse, and ward secretaries. Nursing administration support services are comprised of the director of nursing, associate directors, in-service educators, shift supervisors, infection control coordinator, nursing staff office secretary, and staffing office personnel (see Figure 5-4). Tables 5-1 and 5-2 show a method for determining the cost of these two services.

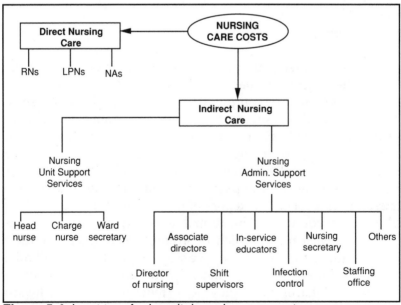

Figure 5-4. Input tree for hospital nursing care costs.

Table 5-1. Method to determine nursing unit support services cost.

Nursing Unit Personnel	Annual Salary	Benefits	Coverage	Total
1. Head nurse	X_1	X_2	X_3	TX_i
2. Charge nurse e.g., extra $0.5/hr. @ 1950 hrs/yr.	Y_1	--	--	Y_i
3. Ward secretaries - Day clerks	D_1	D_2	D_3	TD_i
- Evening clerks	E_1	E_2	E_3	TE_i
				Total = Z
Therefore, $Z = TX_i + Y_i + TD_i + TE_i$ dollars per year Nursing unit support services cost per patient day = Z/Total patient days per year				

Direct nursing care costs consist of the following three components:

- salaries
- benefits
- coverage

The total nursing unit labor cost per hour is stated as the sum of the average of salary, benefits, and coverage cost.

Salaries should be computed with a weighted average since the staff for each nursing unit is comprised of a mixture of skill levels. For example, if a nursing unit maintains a staff size of 10 nurses per day, consisting of five RNs, three LPNs, and two NAs, then 50% of the team is RNs, 30% LPNs, and 20% NAs. A weighted average hourly pay is then computed using the average salary rate for each category of nursing staff. This procedure takes into account the educational level, experience, and competence of each nurse which is, in general, reflected by their salaries, and is the least subjective way of quantifying skill mix.

Employment benefits usually include social security (employer's share), unemployment (federal and state), health and life insurance (employer's share), disability, and worker's

Table 5-2. Method to determine nursing administration support services cost.

Nursing Administration Personnel	Annual Salary	Benefits	Total
1. Director of nursing	A_1	A_2	TA_i
2. Associate directors			
I	B_1	B_2	TB_i
II	C_1	C_2	TC_i
3. In Service educators			
Instructor I	D_1	D_2	TD_i
Instructor II	E_1	E_2	TE_i
Instructor III	F_1	F_2	TF_i
Secretary	G_1	G_2	TG_i
4. Infection control coordinator	H_1	H_2	TH_i
5. Nursing office secretarial staff	I_1	I_2	TI_i
6. Staffing office personnel			
Staffing I	J_1	J_2	TJ_i
Staffing II	K_1	K_2	TK_i
7. Shift supervisors			
Shift I	L_1	L_2	TL_i
Shift II	M_1	M_2	TM_i
Shift III	N_1	N_2	TN_i
			Total = W

where, $W = TA_i + TB_i + \ldots + TN_i$ dollars per year and
$\quad TA_i = A_1 + A_2$;
$\quad\quad TB_i = B_1 + B_2$; etc.
Nursing admin. support services cost per patient day = W/Total patient days

compensation (employer's share). Each benefit is expressed as a percentage of average salary.

Because hospitals are seven-days-a-week enterprises, the cost of employee absences, such as holidays, vacations, training, and sick days, must be covered. Coverage costs are typically expressed in terms of average days per employee per year. The sum of average employee absences per year is stated as a percent of total working days in the year. Coverage cost is stated as a percent of average pay (salaries plus benefits).

Non-nursing care costs are those costs that are traditionally separate from direct nursing. These costs are being considered here because they are traceable to patients in a given nursing unit. Non-nursing costs include room and bed (physical only), ancillary costs, and overhead costs. Traditionally, room and bed costs have included nursing care costs, depreciation, and interest on buildings, capital related to equipment, maintenance and repairs, operation of plant, laundry and linen, dietary, administrative and general, and housekeeping. A step is taken here to untangle the cost of nursing from the cost of room and bed. For our purposes, the cost of room and bed will be the cost of the physical facility only, consisting of the following:

- depreciation, interest on buildings, and fixed capital
- capital related to the equipment
- maintenance and repairs
- operation of plant
- laundry and linen
- housekeeping

Table 5-3 shows a method for determining unit-based non-nursing care costs.

Ancillary costs include supplies, drugs, x-rays, radiology, EKG, EEG, etc. Table 5-4 shows a method for determining the average ancillary cost.

Overhead costs consist of the following: administration (admitting, billing, etc.), dietary, cafeteria, medical records, social services, and miscellaneous. Table 5-5 shows a method for determining overhead costs. The total fixed overhead cost will be the sum of items 2 and 4. The variable cost is expressed as a function of total patient days in the nursing units, whereas fixed cost is a function of admissions. Other criteria may also be utilized in making the distinction between variable and fixed overhead, depending on a hospital's cost allocation system.

Table 5-3. How to determine unit-based non-nursing care costs.

Serial Costs	Room & Bed Overhead Costs	Serial Ancillary Costs
1. Depreciation and interest on buildings and fixtures	1. Radiology	1. Administrative and general (billing, admitting, etc.)
2. Capital related to major movers	2. Supplies	2. Dietary
3. Maintenance and repairs	3. Drugs (pharmacy)	3. Cafeteria
4. Operating of plant	4. X-rays	4. Medical records
5. Laundry and linen	5. EKG	5. Social services
6. Housekeeping	6. EEG	6. Miscellaneous
	7. Others	
Average room and bed cost per patient day = sum of room and bed costs (1 through 6)/total patient days		

Table 5-4. How to determine average ancillary cost.

DRG#	Number of Patients	Total Ancillary Charges	Average Ancillary per DRG
1.	N_1	T_1	T_1/N_1
2.	N_2	T_2	T_2/N_2
3.	N_3	T_3	T_3/N_3
--	--	--	--
490.	N_{490}	T_{490}	T_{490}/N_{490}

Table 5-5. How to determine overhead costs.

Overhead Costs Elements	Fixed	Variable
1. Administrative and general (billing, admitting, etc.)	X	
2. Dietary		X
3. Cafeteria	X	
4. Medical records		X
5. Social services	X	
6. Miscellaneous	X	

While the structure presented in the input tree (Figure 5-5) may not be applicable in all cases, it provides a general and systematic procedure for studying cost components for many types of hospitals. Any meaningful step towards cost containment must begin with an understanding of cost components, their constituencies (discussed in this chapter), and the major cost driver.

A CASE EXAMPLE

Two hospital medical-surgical units were studied for six months. The following is a case example of applying the productivity measurement model discussed above to the two units. First, the input values for each unit will be calculated and explained. Then they will be combined in Tables 5-6 through 5-9 for the total productivity analysis.

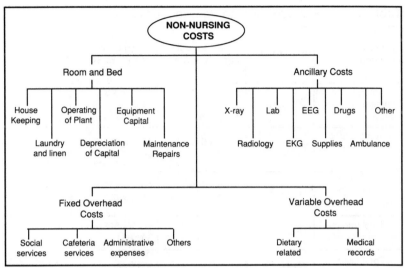

Figure 5-5. Input tree for hospital non-nursing care costs.

1. Total patient days (TPD).

a) The total patient days (actual) per unit per study period represents the sum of all patient days per unit per study period = 5100.

b) The total patient days (standard) in unit A represents the sum of the DRG-based government prescribed patient days for all patients admitted and treated in unit A during the period = 4027.

Hence, the government's prescribed patient days for the types of patients admitted to the unit was 21% less than the actual. The corresponding actual and standard total patient days for unit B are 6458 and 4561. Again, the patient difference in the case of unit B is 29.4%.

2. Average hours of care per patient day (H).
The value for the average hours of care per patient day can be determined from a patient classification system. Most patient classification systems are used to allocate points to patients according to acuity and the ability of patients to function independently. The acuity

Table 5-6. Total productivity analysis for unit A.

Productivity Elements	Equations	Using Actual Length of Stay	Using Standard Length of Stay
1. Total direct nursing care costs	TPD x H x Y	5100 x 4.8 x $13.34 = $326,563	4027 x 4.8 x 13.34 = $257,857
2. Total indirect nursing care costs	TPD x INC	5100 x $1687 = $86,037	4027 x $16.87 = $67,935
3. Total room & bed physical costs	TPD x R	5100 x $29 = $147,900	4027 x $16.87 = $116,783
4. Total variable overhead costs	TPD x VOH	5100 x $2460 = $125,460	4027 x $29 = $99,064
5. Total fixed overhead costs	FOH	$71,226	$71,226
6. Total ancillary costs	A	$711,695	$711,695
7. Total nursing unit input	Sum of #1 through #6	$1,468,881	$1,324,561
8. Total nursing unit output	DAD	$1,594,160	$1,594,160
9. Total nursing unit productivity	#8/#7	1.09	1.20
10. Nursing unit quality score*	Q	83%	83%
11. Quality adjusted productivity (QAP)	Q x #9	0.90	1.00
12. Partial productivity (ancillary)	#8/#6	2.24	2.24
13. Partial productivity (overhead)	#8/(#4 + #5)	9.11	9.36
14. Partial Productivity (nursing)	#8/(#1 + #2)	3.86	4.89

* Unit quality score is based on the result derived from a quality measurement instrument administered periodically at the nursing unit. Such an instrument should consider both the JCAHO and the patient-based requirements.

points are subsequently converted to required nursing care hours per patient day. The required hours per patient day can be determined as the ratio of total acuity point divided by the unit census. More efficient methods currently exist in certain hospitals for arriving at the average hours per patient day. For this case example, the average hours per patient day during the study period is given as 4.8 hours per patient day for unit A, and 4.7 hours per patient day for unit B.

3. Cost of direct nursing care per hour (Y).

a) Average hourly nursing salary:
percentage of RNs in 24 hours = 58%
percentage of LPNs in 24 hours = 21%
percentage of NAs in 24 hours = 21%
average RN rate per hour = $10.83
average LPN rate per hour = $8.62
average NA rate per hour = $7.25

Average hourly nursing salary = 10.83(0.58) + 8.62(0.21) + 7.25(0.21)/1.00
= $9.614/hour

Similar calculations produce the value of $9.11/hour for unit B.

b) Benefits. Employment benefits equal 19.6% of the average salary.

Benefits = 0.196 x 9.614
= 1.88/hour

Similar calculations yield a value of $1.79/hour for unit B.

c) Coverage cost. The average employee absence per year is determined as a percentage of total working days, calculated as 16%.

Coverage cost @ 16% of average salary = (9.61 + 1.88) x 0.16
= $1.838/hour

Similar calculations yield a value of $1.75/hour for unit B.

Table 5-7. Total productivity analysis for unit B.

Productivity Elements	Equations	Using Actual Length of Stay	Using Standard Length of Stay
1. Total direct nursing care cost	TPD x H x Y	6458 x 4.7 x $12.65 = $383,960	4561 x 4.7 x 12.6 = $271,174
2. Total indirect nursing care costs	TPD x INC	6458 x $15.41 = $99,518	4561 x $15.41 = $70,285
3. Total room & bed physical costs	TPD x R	5100 x $29 = $147,900	4561 x $29 = $116,783
4. Total variable overhead costs	TPD x VOH	6458 x $24.10 = $155,638	4561 x $24.10 = $107,510
5. Total fixed overhead costs	FOH	$85,781	$85,781
6. Total ancillary costs	A	$999,301	$999,301
7. Total nursing unit input	Sum of #1 through #6	$1,911,480	$1,666,320
8. Total nursing unit output	DAD	$2,049,379	$2,049,379
9. Total nursing unit productivity	#8/#7	1.07	1.23
10. Nursing unit quality score	Q	73%	73%
11. Quality adjusted productivity (QAP)	Q x #9	0.78	0.90
12. Partial productivity (Ancillary)	#8/#6	2.05	2.05
13. Partial productivity (Overhead)	#8/(#4 + #5)	8.49	10.60
14. Partial productivity (Nursing)	#8/(#1 + #2)	4.24	5.00

d) Total direct nursing care cost = $9.61 + $1.88 + $1.84 = $13.34/hour

Similar calculations yield a value of $12.65/hour for unit B.

4. Total indirect nursing costs. Indirect nursing costs (INC) are given as the product of the total patient days in a given unit and

Table 5-8. Nursing productivity analysis for unit A.

Productivity Elements	Equations	Using Actual Length of Stay	Using Standard Length of Stay
1. Total Direct Nursing Care Costs	TPD x H x Y	5100 x 4.8 x $13.34 = $326,563	4027 x 4.8 x 13.34 = $257,857
2. Total Indirect Nursing Care Costs	TPD x INC	5100 x $16.87 = $86,037	4027 x $16.87 = $67,935
3. Total Nursing Unit Input	#1 + #2	$412,600	$325,792
4. Nursing Care Cost at fraction of total	0.281	0.281	0.281
5. Total Nursing Unit Output	DAD	$1,594,160	$1,594,160
6. Total Nursing Unit Productivity	(#5 x #4)/#3	1.09	1.37
7. Nursing Unit Quality Score	83%	83%	83%
8. Quality Adjusted Productivity (QAP)	#6 x #7	0.90	1.14

the indirect nursing care cost per patient day. (Recall that the total indirect nursing care cost is made up of nursing unit support services cost and nursing administration support services cost.) The units A and B figures for the two cost components are shown in Tables 5-10 through 5-12.

5. Room and bed costs (physical). There are several cost accounting systems that can be used to untangle the cost of nursing from the cost of room and bed. The method used in Table 5-13 is chosen only for computational convenience. The analysis includes only the physical costs for room and bed and is based on the total expenses during the study period for units A ($538,161) and B($648,134).

Table 5-9. Nursing productivity analysis for unit B.

Productivity Elements	Equations	Using Actual Length of Stay	Using Standard Length of Stay
1. Total direct nursing	TPD x H x Y	6458 x 4.7 x $12.65 = $383,960	4561 x 4.7 x $12.65 = $271,174
2. Total indirect nursing	TPD x INC	6458 x $15.41 = $99,518	4561 x $15.41 = $71,285
3. Total nursing input	#1 + #2	$483,478	$341,459
4. Nursing cost care as a fraction of total		0.281	0.281
5. Total nursing output	DAD	$2,049,379	$2,049,379
6. Total nursing productivity	(#5 x #4)/#3	1.19	1.69
7. Nursing unit quality score		73%	73%
8. Quality adjusted productivity (QAP)	#6 + #7	0.87	1.23

6. Overhead costs. Two types of overhead costs, variable and fixed, are identified in Figure 5-6. Tables 5-14 and 5-15 present estimates of overhead costs for units A and B during the study period. Recall that the total annual expenses for units A and B are given as $538,161 and $648,134 respectively.

Since the variable overhead cost is a function of patient days, the figures for each unit are divided by the total patient days in the unit.

1) variable overhead cost per patient day (unit A) = $231,947 per year/9,425 patient days per year
= $24.60/patient day

2) variable overhead cost per patient day (unit B) = $279,346 per year/11,606 patient days per year
= $24.10/patient day

Table 5-10. Nursing unit support services unit A.

	Annual Salary	Benefits (@ 19.6%)	Coverage	Total
Head nurse	$25,623	$5,022	0	$30,645
Charge nurse (extra $0.5/hr) @ 1950 hrs/yr.)	$975	0	0	$975
Ward secretaries(day or unit clerk) 1 day @ $7.90/hr 1 day @ $8.57/hr	$15,405 $16,712	$3,019 $3,276	$2,392 $2,598	$20,819 $22,585
			Annual total	$75,025

Note: Benefits = 19.6% of average salary
      Coverage = approximately 16% of average salary
Total patient days for the year in unit A = 9,425

Nursing unit support for unit A = $75,025/9,425
                   = $7.96/patient day

Since the study period was six months (one half year), the estimated fixed overhead costs for units A and B are $71,226 ($142,451/2), and $85,781 ($171,562/2), respectively.

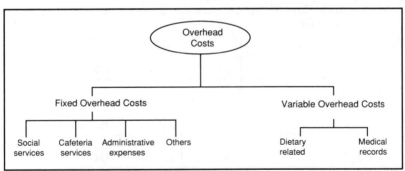

Figure 5-6. A breakdown of overhead costs.

7. Ancillary cost. The total ancillary cost of a nursing unit should be adjusted to include the associated indirect costs. Suppose that the total ancillary cost is $711,696 for unit A and $999,300 for unit B. These costs are for the study period.

Table 5-11. Nursing administration support services (for the hospital).

	Annual Salary	Benefits	Total
Director of nursing	$43,000	$8,428	$51,428
Associate director of nursing (2 persons)	a) $31,883	$6,249	$38,132
	b) $31,883	$6,249	$38,132
In-service educators	$31,883	$6,249	$38,132
a) Instructor I	$25,064	$4,913	$29,977
b) Instructor II	$24,616	$4,825	$29,977
c) Instructor P/T	$14,916	$2,924	$17,840
d) Secretary	$16,444	$3,223	$19,667
Infection control coordinator	$24,951	$4,890	$29,841
Nursing office secretarial staff	$17,589	$3,447	$21,036
Staffing office personnel (2 persons)	a) $17,589	$3,363	$20,523
	b) $16,478	$3,229	$19,707
Shift supervisor			
a) Shift 1	$28,919	$5,668	$34,587
b) Shift 2	$26,000	$5,096	$31,096
c) Shift 3	$15.68/hr	0	0
		Annual Total	$419,529

Note: Benefits = 19.6% of average salary
Nursing administration support services for unit A (where total patient days for the hospital per year = 47,100) = $419,539/47,100
= $8.91/patient day (Hospital-wide)
Total indirect nursing care cost/patient day = $7.96 + $8.91
= $16.87 per patient day

Table 5-12. Nursing unit support services.

	Total	Annual Salary	Benefits (@ 19.6%)	Coverage
Head nurse	$25,955	$5,087	0	$31,042
Charge nurse (extra $0.50/hr @ 1950 hrs/yr)	$975	0	0	$975
Ward secretaries (day or unit clerk)				
1 day @ $7.90/hr	$15,405	$3,019	$2,392	$20,819
1 day @ $8.57/hr	$16,712	$3,276	$2,598	$22,585
				Total $75,425

Note: Benefits = 19.6% of averge salary
      Coverage = approximately 16.1% of average salary
Total patient days for the year in unit B = 11,606 (1985)
Nursing administration support services for unit B = $75,422/11,606
                                      = $6.50/patient day
Recall that nursing administration support services for the hospital was given as $8.91/patient day.
Total indirect nursing care cost/patient day = $6.50 + $8.91
                                      = $15.41 per patient day

8. DRG Revenue. Suppose we define the total output of the nursing unit as the sum of all DRG amounts due for all patients in the unit during the study period. The figures are $1,594,160 for unit A and $2,049,379 for unit B.

The data needed for productivity computations for units A and B are summarized in Table 5-16.

Analysis of Results

Table 5-17 gives a summary of the productivity analysis presented earlier in this chapter. Each value in the table is discussed below.

Table 5-13. Room and bed (physical) for units A and B.

Cost Components	Percent of total expenses*	Unit A	Unit B
1. Depreciation and interest on buildings and other fixed assets	5.1%	$ 27,466	$ 33,055
2. Capital related to major movers--depreciation and interest related to movable equipment	0.73%	$ 3,929	$ 4,731
3. Maintenance and repairs	7.20%	$ 38,748	$ 46,666
4. Plant operation	19.30%	$103,865	$125,090
5. Laundry and linen	5.40%	$ 29,061	$ 34,999
6. Housekeeping	13.60%	$ 73,190	$ 88,146
Total per year		$ 27,239	$332,687

* Percentages can be estimated from historical data or from a budget breakdown. The cost components may also be different from one facility to another.
a) Room and bed cost per patient day (unit A) = $276,239 per year/9,425 patients for the year = $29 per patient day
b) Similarly, room and bed cost per patient day (unit B) = $332,687/11,606 = $29 per patient day

1. Total productivity. The total productivity of a nursing unit has been defined as the ratio of the total output (in terms of DRG revenues generated by the patients admitted to the unit) to the total input (all resources—human and non-human resources consumed in treating patients). This ratio is calculated using a actual length of stay (LOS) and the government prescribed or standard length of stay. The respective values for nursing unit A are 1.09 and 1.20 (a difference of 10%), and for B, 1.07 and 1.23 (a difference of 15%). Since units A and B are both medical-surgical units, a within-hospital comparison can be made. These results show that for every dollar of health-care cost within unit A, the hospital generates $1.09 in revenues, and for unit B it generates $1.07 in revenues. Two other important points should be made from these results. First, the disparity between the

Table 5-14. Variable overhead cost for units A and B.

Variable Overhead Cost Components	Percent of Total Expenses	Unit A	Unit B
1. Dietary	34.9%	$187,818	$226,199
2. Medical records and library	8.20%	$ 44,129	$ 53,147
Total		$231,947	$279,346

Table 5-15. Fixed overhead cost for units A and B.

Fixed Overhead Cost Components	Percent of Total Expenses	Unit A	Unit B
1. Administration & general overhead	19.8%	$106,555	$128,331
2. Cafeteria	3.60%	$19,372	$23,333
3. Central services	0.13%	$700	$843
4. Pharmacy	0.14%	$753	$907
5. Social services	2.80%	$15,069	$18,148
Total fixed overhead cost/year		$142,451	$171,562

actual and the prescribed length of stay would be studied for its effect on productivity. Second, although both units are medical-surgical units, and therefore admit and treat similar patients, unit A departs less from the prescribed length of stay. Comparatively, it seems slightly more cost-efficient to treat patients in unit B than A. From the analysis, unit B shows a slightly more efficient use of resources.

Table 5-16. Data summary.

	Unit A	Unit B
a) Total patient days	5100	6458
b) Nursing hours per patient day	4.8	4.7
c) Total direct nursing care cost per hour	$13.34	$12.65
d) Total indirect nursing care cost per patient day	$16.87	$15.41
e) Average room and bed cost per patient day	$29.60	$29.00
f) Variable overhead cost per patient day	$24.60	$24.10
g) Fixed overhead cost per study period	$71,226	$85,785

2. *Quality adjusted productivity.* Quality scores are determined
from an instrument designed to capture the degree to which a
nursing unit complies with JCAHO's standard, as well as the
degree to which customer requirements are met. The scores
used in this example are derived from the scores developed
from the Rush-Medicus quality instrument. Although only a
handful of instruments exists that include customer-based requirements, there appears to be some movement towards incor-
porating patient requirements in new instruments. With quality
scores of 83% and 73% respectively for units A and B, the
quality adjusted productivity (QAP) for unit A is higher than
that of B.

Table 5-17. Summary of productivity analysis (unit and nursing-based productivity).

	Unit A n = 5100 pt. days		Unit B n = 6458 pt. days	
	Actual LOS	Standard LOS	Actual LOS	Standard LOS
1. Total productivity of nursing unit (UBA)	1.09	1.20	1.07	1.23
2. Quality adjusted productivity	0.90	1.00	0.78	0.98
3. Partial productivity (Ancillary)	2.24	2.24	2.05	2.05
4. Partial productivity * (Overhead)	8.11	9.36	8.50	10.60
5. Partial productivity (Nursing)	3.86	4.90	4.24	6.02
6. Total productivity of nursing in the unit (UBA)	1.09	1.37	1.20	1.69
7. Total productivity of the unit (UBA), 3rd quarter	1.06	1.22	1.01	1.19
8. Total productivity of units (UBA), 4th quarter	1.12	1.21	1.06	1.22
9. Productivity of nursing (NBA), 3rd quarter	1.04	1.39	1.13	1.74
10. Productivity of nursing (NBA), 4th quarter	1.16	1.38	1.16	1.67

*Partial productivity is not used in its traditional sense here, since labor and material costs are not included.

One of the advantages of integrating quality scores with productivity measures is that it emphasizes the need to attain lower cost without compromising the standard of care. Although most hospital quality assurance programs are somewhat subjective, a shift towards quantifiable measures will minimize the subjectivity over time. If a hospital is able to develop a quality monitoring measure based on compliance to the requirements of the Joint Commission and a measure of the degree to which customers' expectations are met, such measures can be used to generate quality scores. Issues addressed in these measures include the friendliness of nurses, ability to effectively answer patients' questions, ability to answer physicians' questions, food quality, etc.

3. Partial productivity. The essence of a partial productivity measure lies in its ability to determine the changes in the value of output against changes in any one class of input. In the case of the ancillary value, the ratio of revenue to the dollar value of ancillary for the study period was 2.24 for unit A, and 2.05 for unit B. This ratio reveals that unit A spends less on ancillary costs than unit B. Another way of stating this is that unit A spends $1.00 on ancillary costs for every $2.24 of revenues generated by the unit; unit B spends $1.00 for every $2.05 of revenues.

This partial (ancillary) productivity ratio is a mechanism for monitoring ancillary resource consumption over time and its subsequent effect on total productivity. Each partial measure indicates savings achieved over time in each of the inputs per output unit. Partial measures can be used as planning tools from period to period. The figures for the partial productivity of overhead show that for unit A, one dollar of overhead expense equals $8.11 of revenues generated by the unit during the study period. Similarly, for unit B, one dollar of overhead expense is equivalent to $8.50 in revenues. Since nursing is one of the most important factors in a unit, the partial productivity measure is essential with respect to nursing. For units A and B, each dollar of nursing resources is equivalent to $3.86 and $4.24 of revenues generated by the unit during the study period.

It is the concern of nursing and hospital management to monitor changes in these ratios from one period to another and to use them for planning. Partial measures can help nursing management identify which resource consumption needs better management and which has the greatest impact on the total productivity of the unit.

4. Productivity with respect to nursing. Nursing unit productivity is the ratio of the dollar value of nursing intervention revenues to the dollar value of nursing care cost. The figures are $1.09 and $1.20 for units A and B respectively. The total revenue generated by patients admitted to each unit is adjusted by the ratio of total cost of nursing to the total expenses of the hospital. This represents a hospital-wide ratio applied to each unit. This adjustment factor can be a starting point for research on the proportion of revenues attributed to nursing intervention. This ratio is 28.1% for the hospital studied. Total nursing care cost is the cost for direct and indirect nursing care (including administrative and all nursing division personnel). Estimated revenues attributable to nursing are found by multiplying 28.1% (the adjustment factor) by the total revenue. If a more accurate figure is available to figure nursing related revenues, it should be used. Therefore, it can be stated that for every dollar of nursing cost expended in units A and B, revenues of $1.09 and $1.20, respectively, are generated. The total productivity for unit A is found to be consistently higher than that of unit B during the third and fourth quarters of the year. On the other hand, the productivity of nursing is higher in the third quarter for unit B.

Diagnosis-Based Productivity

The analyses presented next are based on selected DRGs in the hospital studied. The diagnoses selected for productivity analysis are DRGs 127, 140, 089, 096, 182, and 294. A brief description of the selected DRGs are presented in Table 5-18.

Diagnosis-Based Productivity Calculation

Table 5-19 shows the computation for diagnosis-based productivity values for a DRG from each unit. Summaries of the results for the six DRGs studied are presented in Tables 5-20 and 5-21, for units A and B respectively.

Table 5-18. DRG descriptions.

DRG	Description
127	Acute and/or subacute endocarditis
140	Angina
089	Simple Pneumonia and/or pleurisy (Patients who are over age 70 and/or have a substantial complication or comorbidity.)
096	Bronchitis and/or Asthma (Patients who are over age 70 and/or have a substantial complication or comorbidity.)
182	Gastrointestinal disorder (Patients who are over age 70 and/or have a substantial complicatin or comorbidity.)
294	Diabetes, age 36+

The following observations can be made from the above calculations:

• For every dollar of total resources consumed in treating patients of DRG 127, unit A generates a revenue of $0.97, while unit B generates a revenue of $1.09.

• Similarly, for DRG 089, unit A generates $1.11 in revenues for every dollar of resources consumed, while unit B loses eight cents for every dollar of resource consumption.

• Unit B appears to be more efficient than unit A in treatment of DRG 294 patients. Unit B generates a revenue of $1.66 per dollar of resources to $0.94 of unit A.

Although longer LOS corresponds to higher resource consumption, the rate of consumption towards the end of hospitalization is not as high as the rate at the beginning of hospitalization. The relationship between LOS and resource

Table 5-19. An example of diagnosis-based productivity analysis.

	Unit A	Unit B
	DRG 089	**DRG 127**
1. Number of patients	14	84
2. Total patient days	161	943
3. Average LOS	11.5	11.23
4. Direct nursing care costs	161 x H x Y = $10,309	943 x H x Y = $56,066
5. Indirect nursing care costs	161 x $16.87 = $2,716	943 x $15.41 = $14,532
6. Total room & bed costs	161 x $29 = $4,669	943 x $29 = $27,347
7. Total variable overhead costs	161 x $24.60 = $3,961	943 x $24.10 = $22,726
8. Diagnosis patient days/Total patient days	161/5100 = 0.0316	943/6458 = 0.146
9. Total fixed overhead cost	$71,226 x #8 = $2,249	$85,781 x #8 = $12,52
10. Total diagnosis ancillary cost	$22,432	$114,209
11. Total diagnosis-based output	Sum of #s 4, 5, 6, 7, 9, and 10 = $46,336	Sum of #s 4, 5, 6, 7, 9, and 10 = $247,406
12. Total diagnosis-based output	$51,606	$261,113
13. Diagnosis-based productivity	#12/#11 = 1.11	#12/#11 = 1.06
14. Unit quality score	83%	73%
15. Quality adjusted productivity	#13 x #14 = 0.92	#13 x #14 = 0.77

Table 5-20. Summary of diagnosis-based productivity analysis (unit A).

Variables	DRG Number					
	127	140	089	096	182	294
Number of patients	13	3	14	5	15	8
Total patient days	130	16	161	26	126	68
Average LOS	10.0	5.3	11.5	5.2	8.4	8.5
Prescribed LOS	9.10	6.90	10.50	8.03	6.80	8.90
Diagnosis specific productivity	0.97	1.26	1.11	1.39	0.90	0.94

consumption is supported by the fact that in all six DRG cases selected, the shorter the average LOS, the higher the corresponding value of the diagnosis-related productivity for the hospital. This shows that there is a significant relationship between LOS and resource consumption and also between LOS and productivity.

The productivity measurement approaches described above are not without their limitations. The volume and types of information needed to ensure the success of the approaches make the management of productivity very challenging. It would be very tedious to handle this magnitude of information manually. The approaches, however, lend themselves to spreadsheet and other software applications. The economics of today's healthcare environment dictate that we pay greater attention to costs than we have in the past. This three-part model of hospital productivity can be integrated into a hospital's cost accounting system.

Table 5-21. Summary of diagnosis-based productivity analysis (unit B).

	DRG Number					
Variables	**127**	**140**	**089**	**096**	**182**	**294**
Number of patients	82	90	6	5	11	2
Total patient days	807	568	173	73	54	12
Average LOS	9.80	6.31	28.80	14.60	4.90	6.00
Prescribed LOS	9.10	6.90	10.50	8.03	6.80	8.90
Diagnosis specific productivity	1.09	1.25	0.92	0.88	1.97	1.66

OTHER MEASUREMENT MODELS

Although several models have been proposed for the measurement of productivity in health care, very few of them lend themselves to quantification. Among them is a model developed by Benson (1981) and Dennis, Dunn, and Benson (1980).

Dennis, et al. (1980) developed a model to measure the productivity of nursing personnel in an acute care hospital. In his work, input and output are defined as follows:

$$\text{Input} = I = \sum_{i=1}^{3} S_i N_i$$

Where: S_i = the salary ratio of type i nurses
N_i = the number of type i nursing hours worked
i = 1; registered nurse
= 2; licensed practical nurse
= 3; nursing assistant

Output = O = $0.5T_1 + 1T_2 + 2.5T_3 + 5T_4$

Where: T_1 = the number of type 1 patients on a unit
           T_2 = the number of type 2 patients on a unit
           T_3 = the number of type 3 patients on a unit
           T_4 = the number of type 4 patients on a unit

According to Benson, the intensity of care required for the four patient types is approximated by the ratio 0.5:1.0:2.5:5.0. The ratio is based on the definition of type 2 patients as the average in a four-level patient classification system. Benson then defines the productivity index as the ratio of output to input.

Others who have developed quantifiable measures of productivity in health care include Mundel (1983), Jelinek and Dennis (1976), and Curtin and Zurlage (1986). The inefficient use of health-care resources, lack of attention to quality issues, the increasing number of uninsured individuals seeking care, and increased competition, continue to be the main reasons for the declining economic health of health-care organizations. There is a critical need to understand health-care costs and their driving forces. Everyone, especially physicians, must be made aware of the impact of inefficiency in resource utilization, medication errors, delays due to improper procedures, and the time taken to correct errors and mistakes. When these issues go unmanaged, quality is compromised and productivity decreases.

EXERCISES

5-1. What measures of productivity are currently in use at your hospital? In what ways do they differ from the ones presented in this chapter?

5-2. What changes would need to be made to your information management system in order to use the models described in the chapter?

5-3. Conduct a study to determine the distribution of the following resources for a given day of hospitalization. In other words, for a patient whose LOS is five days, what percentagof his/her total ancillary resources was consumed on day 1, day 2, ..., day 5?

- direct nursing care cost
- indirect nursing care cost
- ancillary cost

5-4. What conclusion can you draw regarding the use of these resources towards the beginning and end of hospitalization?

BIBLIOGRAPHY

Adam, Jr., E. E., J. C. Hershauer, and W. A. Ruch. 1981. *Productivity and Quality: Measurement as a Basis for Improvement.* Englewood Cliffs, NJ: Prentice-Hall.

Aggarwal, S. C. 1979. A study of productivity measures for improving benefit-cost ratios of operating operations. Amsterdam, Netherlands: *Proceedings of 5th International Conference on Production Research.* pp. 64-70.

American Hospital Association. 1973. *The Management of Hospital Employee Productivity: An Introductory Handbook.* Chicago: American Hospital Association.

Anderson, M. L. 1980. Productivity monitoring: A key element of productivity. *Cost Containment in Hospitals.* Efraim Turban, ed. Rockville, MD: Aspen Systems Corporation.

Arndt, M. and B. Skydell. 1985. Inpatient nursing services; productivity and cost. *Costing Out Nursing Services: Pricing Our Product.* National League for Nursing. Pub. no. 20-1982. p. 135.

Aydelotte, M. K. 1973. Staffing for high quality care. *Hospitals.* (47)58:60.

Baar, A. 1967. *Measurement of Nursing Care*. Oxford Regional Hospital Board, Operational Research Unit. Pub. no. 9.

Ballard, D., K. B. Barack, and J. J. Cullen. 1985. The variable nursing charge system at the Hospital of Saint Raphael. National League for Nursing. Pub. no. 20-1982.

Bennett, Addison C. 1983. *Productivity and the Quality of Work Life in Hospitals*. Chicago: American Hospital Association.

Benson, G. C. 1981. Model to measure the productivity of nursing personnel in acute care hospitals. *AIIE Annual Conference Proceedings*. Norcross, GA: American Institute of Industrial Engineers. Spring. p. 230.

Bertz, E. J. 1983. Hospital productivity plays key role under prospective pricing. *The Hospital Manager*. Chicago: American Hospital Association. Nov.-Dec.

Buller, B. 1984. Consolidation raises staff productivity. *Hospitals*. 58(17):49-50.

Caterinicchio, R. and R. Davies. 1983. Developing a client focused resource use: An alternative to the patient day. *Social Science and Medicine*. 17:259-272.

Caterinicchio, R. and J. Warren. DRGs and medical practice: Meeting the challenge of incentive reimbursement. *The Journal of the Medical Society of New Jersey*. pp. 895-898.

Cleverly, W. O. 1977. Cost containment in health care industry. *Topics in Health Care Financing*. Rockville, MD: Aspen Systems Corporation.

Coventry, L. 1984. A report on the national invitational conference on nursing productivity. Washington, DC: Georgetown University.

Craig, C. E. and C. R. Harris. 1973. The productivity measurement at the firm level. *Sloan Management Review*. 14(3):13-29.

Curtin, L. L. 1984. Reconciling pay with productivity. *Nursing Management.* 15(2):7.

Curtin, L. L. and C. Zurlage. 1986. Nursing productivity: From data to definition. *Nursing Management.* 17(6):32.

Dahlen, A. L. and J. R. Gregor. 1982. Nursing costs by DRG with an all RN staff. *Costing Out Nursing Services: Pricing Our Product.* National League for Nursing. Pub. no. 20. p. 113.

Dennis, L. C. and R. C. Jelinek. 1976. A review and evaluation of nursing productivity. *Health Manpower References.* DHEW Pub. no. (HRA) 77-15.

Dennis, L. C., M. G. Dunn, and G. C. Benson. 1980. An empirical model for measuring nursing productivity in acute care hosptials. DHHH Contract no. 231-77-0121.

DiVesta, N. 1984. The changing health care system: An overview. *DRGs: Changes and Challenges.* Franklin A. Schaffer, ed. New York: National League for Nursing. Pub. no. 20-1959.

DeWitt, F. 1970. Techniques for measuring productivity. *Management Review.* 59:2-11.

Donabedian, A. 1976. Some basic issues in evaluating the quality of care. *Issues in Evaluation Research.* New York: American Nurses Association. Pub. no. G124M. p. 7.

_____ .1980. The definition of quality and approaches to its assessment. *Explorations in Quality Assurance and Monitoring.* Ann Arbor, MI: Health Administration Press.

Edwardson, R. R. 1985. Measuring nursing productivity. *Nursing Economics.* 3(1):9-14.

Eusebio, E., K. Louisengnau, M. Horger-Scheuber, and J. Jorlett. 1985. Product selection in the hospital: Controlling cost. *Nursing Management.* 16(3):44-46.

Fetter, R. B., Y. Shinn, J. Freeman, R. Averill, et al. 1980. Case mix definition by diagnosis-related groups. *Medical Care.* 18(2): 41-53.

Filley, R. D. 1985. Health care costs take spotlight as technological advances collide with issues and practicalities. *Industrial Engineering.* Norcross, GA: Institute of Industrial Engineers. 17(3):35.

Franz, J. Challenge for nursing: Hiking productivity without lowering quality of care. *Modern Healthcare.* pp.60-68.

Ganong, J. M. and W. L. Ganong. 1984. *Performance Appraisal for Productivity: The Nurse Manager's Handbook.* Rockville, MD: Aspen Systems Corporation.

Giovannetti, P. 1986. A report on the national invitational conference on nursing productivity. Washington, DC: Georgetown University. p. 41.

Graham, N. 1982. *Quality Assurance in Hospitals: Strategies for Assessment and Implementation.* Gaithersburg, MD: Aspen Systems Corporation.

Gray, S. P. and W. Steffy. 1983. *Hospital Cost Containment Through Productivity Management.* New York, NY: Van Nostrand Reinhold Company.

Griffith, J. R. 1978. *Measuring Hospital Performance.* Blue Cross Association.

Haas, S. W. 1984. Sorting out nursing productivity. *Nursing Management.* 15(4):37-40.

Hanson, R. L. 1982. Managing human resources. *Journal of Nursing Administration.* 12(2):17-23.

Haussmann, R. K., S. T. Hegyvary, and J. F. Newman. 1985. Quality of nursing care: Assessment and correlates. Rush-Presbyterian-St. Luke's Medical Center and Medicus Systems Corporation.

Hegyvary, S. T. and R. K. Haussmann. 1976. Correlates of nursing care quality. *Journal of Nursing Administration.* 6(9):22-27.

Herzog, T. P. 1985. Productivity: Fighting the battle of the budget. *Nursing Management.* 16(1):30-34.

Hines, W. W. 1976. Guidelines for implementing productivity measurement. *Industrial Engineering.* Norcross, GA: Institute of Industrial Engineers. 8(6):40-43.

Jelinek, R. C. and L. C. Dennis. 1976. *A Review and Evaluation of Nursing Productivity.* Bethesda, MD: DHEW Pub. no. (HRA) 77-15.

Levine, E. 1984. Some issues in nursing productivity. *Costing Out Nursing: Pricing Our Product.* Franklin A. Schaffer, ed. New York: National League for Nursing. Pub. no. 20-1982. p. 237.

Luke, R. D., J. C. Krueger, and R. E. Modrow. 1984. *Organization and Change in Health Care Quality Assurance.* Rockville, MD: Aspen Publications.

Lewis, E. N. and P. V. Carini. 1984. *Nurse Staffing and Patient Classification.* Rockville, MD: Aspen Publications.

Maraldo, P. J. 1984. The challenge: Health care in crisis. *DRG's Changes and Challenges.* New York: National League for Nursing. Pub. no. 20-1959. p. 9.

Medicus Systems Corporation. 1980. *Productivity and Health: A Review and Evaluation of Health Personnel Productivity.* Hyattsville, MD: U.S. Public Health Service. DHHS Pub. no. (HRA) 80-14029.

Meyer, D. 1985. Costing nursing care with the GRASP system. *Costing Out Nursing: Pricing Our Product.* Franklin A. Shaffer, ed. New York: National League for Nursing. Pub. no. 20-1982.

Millenson, M. L. 1987. A prescription for change. *Quality Progress.* 20(5):18.

Mitchell, M., J. Miller, J. Welches, and D. Walker. 1984. Determining cost of direct nursing care by DRGs. *Nursing Management.* 15(4).

Mundel, M. E. 1983. *Improving Productivity and Effectiveness.* Englewood Cliffs, NJ: Prentice Hall International Series in Industrial and Systems Engineering.

Nadler, G. and V. Sahney. 1969. A descriptive model of nursing care. *American Journal of Nursing.* 69:336-341.

Nunamaker, T. R. 1983. Measuring routine nursing service efficiency: A comparison of cost per patient day and data envelopment analysis model. *Health Services Research.* 18(2).

Omachonu, V. K. and R. Nanda. 1988. Hospital nursing unit productivity measurement: A conceptual framework. *Industrial Engineering.* Norcross, GA: Institute of Industrial Engineers. 20(5):56.

_____. 1988. Developing an information base for measuring nursing unit productivity. *Institute of Industrial Engineers Fall Conference Proceedings,* Norcross, GA: Institute of Industrial Engineers.

_____. 1988. Diagnosis-based approach to hospital nursing unit productivity measurement. *Proceedings of the Ninth Annual Conference, American Society for Engineering Management.* Knoxville, TN: American Society for Engineering Management.

_____. 1989. Measuring productivity: Outcome vs. output. *Nursing Management.* 20(4):35.

_____.1989. Measuring hospital nursing unit productivity under the new reimbursement system. *Productivity Management Frontiers II.* D. S. Sumanth, et al., ed. Switzerland: Inderscience Enterprises, Ltd. p. 63.

_____. 1990. Model-based hospital productivity information management. *Journal of Computers and Industrial Engineering.*

Omachonu, V. K., E. A. Sorrentino, and E. Worley. 1990. Management implications of DRGs in hospitals. *Journal of Health and Human Resources.*

Richards, G. 1983. Working smarter-productivity takes on new importance under prospective pricing. *Hospitals.* p.92.

Riley, W. J.and V. Schaefers. 1983. Costing nursing services. *Nursing Management.* 14:40-43.

_____. 1984. Nursing operations as profit center. *Nursing Management.* 15(4):43.

Ryan, J. 1987. Health care quality assurance regulation. *Quality Progress.* 20(5):27.

Schroeder, P. and R. Mailbusch. 1984. *Nursing Quality Assurance: A Unit-Based Approach.* Gaithersburg, MD: Aspen Systems Corporation.

Sink, D. S. 1985. *Productivity Management: Planning, Measurement and Evaluation, Control and Improvement.* New York: John Wiley & Sons.

Smalley, H. E. 1982. *Hospital Management Engineering.* Englewood Cliffs, NJ: Prentice Hall International Series on Industrial and Systems Engineering.

Sumanth, D. J. 1984. *Productivity Engineering and Management.* New York: McGraw-Hill Book Company.

Toth, R. M. 1984. *DRGs as a Power Base for Nursing Service Administration.* National League for Nursing. Pub. no. 20-1959.

Walker, D. 1983. The cost of nursing care in hospitals. *Journal of Nursing Administration.* 13:13-18.

Ziegenfuss, Jr., J. T. 1985. *DRGs and Hospital Impact*. New York: McGraw-Hill Book Company.

6 Managing Productivity, Profitability, and Price Recovery

The era of indiscriminate use of health-care resources is behind us. Today, health-care organizations are preoccupied with the challenge of monitoring resource consumption while delivering care effectively and efficiently. Traditionally, concerns over profitability and price recovery were expressed only by budget directors, hospital accountants, and administrators. Treating each of the 490 Diagnosis Related Groups (DRGs) as a product line opens up some interesting possibilities for cost accounting analysis. Each DRG can now be scrutinized for profitability, productivity, and price recovery.

Monitoring the level of productivity in a hospital's unit is an important management function, especially if the hospital is to remain competitive in today's marketplace. The Multi-Factor Productivity Measurement Model (MFPMM) is one method for managing the productivity of a hospital unit (Sink 1985). This procedure is based on the premise that a firm generates profits from two sources: productivity and price recovery improvement. Productivity is used here as a measure of real growth changes in physical input and output quantities. Price recovery is the extent to which input cost or price increases are passed on to the customers (i.e., the extent to which inflation is recovered through increases in sales price). Since arbitrary price increases cannot be made under a Prospective Pricing System (PPS) reimbursement, price recovery analysis is an effective planning tool for unit managers.

The MFPMM is a dynamic approach for monitoring the productivity of a nursing unit. It relies on general accounting data for costs and revenues. Productivity and price recovery measures pinpoint factors directly influencing profitability at the unit level, e.g., direct nursing care, indirect nursing care, ancillary costs, room and bed costs, and overhead costs. The model compares data from a base period with current period data to generate price quantity and value-weighted change ratios (percentages) from period to period. Thus, it identifies cost drivers for productivity improvement (cost reduction).

The input data required for the MFPMM are periodic for quantity and price. The value data of each input and output are generated by multiplying quantity by price. Depending on an organization's data and record-keeping system, the information needed for MFPMM can be monthly, quarterly, or annually. The model is dynamic in that it compares data from one period (base period) with data from a second period (current or measurement period). This comparison forms the basis of the productivity-price recovery-profitability analysis.

The selection of a base period is critical to the success of this process. A base period is a reference period, a period against which the current or measurement period will be compared. The base period should be a period of normal business activity, with no unusual occurrences or disruptions. In some cases, the base period is selected on the basis of the availability of data to match the current or measurement period.

APPLYING MFPMM TO A HOSPITAL'S NURSING UNIT

A model for measuring the productivity of a nursing unit was presented in Chapter Five. The model defined productivity in the context of DRG revenues and input costs for all resources consumed in treating a patient. A hospital's nursing unit represents the focal point of resource consumption for inpatients. The ability to trace resource consumption to individual patients in a given nursing unit is essential in the management of productivity, profitability, and price recovery, under a prospective payment reimbursement system.

MFPMM is driven by essentially the same accounting data that was used in Chapter Five to track a hospital's revenue and costs. It is a potent diagnostic tool for pointing out the direction for improvement.

The key benefits of applying the MFPMM to a hospital are:

1. Changes in productivity, price recovery, and profitability can be tracked over time for each DRG and nursing unit.

2. Nursing managers and hospital administrators can test "what if" scenarios (in terms of resource consumption).

3. Partial factor productivity ratios can be generated.

4. Challenge budgets for nursing units can be developed.

5. Nursing and hospital administrators can analyze cost drivers.

The driving relationship behind MFPMM is that profitability is a function of productivity and price recovery. Productivity refers to the ratio of quantities of output to quantities of input; price recovery refers to the ratio of prices of output to costs of inputs.

A Case Study Example
The data presented in this example are based on the study of the medical-surgical unit of the general hospital discussed in chapter five. Six months of data were gathered for three selected diagnoses (endocarditis, DRG 127; bronchitis or asthma, DRG 096; and pneumonia or pleurisy, DRG 089). The data were divided into two quarters, with the first quarter selected as the base period. It is also possible to perform this study using semi-annual or annual data depending on the ease of data availability and the purpose for which the analysis is needed. Annual data are more suitable if seasonality is a factor among the selected DRGs. Table 6-1 shows the basic information for this example.

Table 6-1. Basic information for example case study.

DRG name	DRG number	Number of patients in First Quarter (Base period)	Number of patients in Second Quarter (Current period)
1. Acute and/or subacute endocarditis	127	6	7
2. Bronchitis and/or asthma	096	2	3
3. Simple pneumonia and/or pleurisy	089	8	6

As shown in Table 6-1, the numbers of patients treated for diagnoses #127, 096, and 089 during the first quarter were 6, 2, and 8, respectively. Similarly, the corresponding numbers of patients treated in the current period were 7, 3, and 6, respectively.

The computations in Table 6-2 represent the process of deriving the productivity, profitability, and price recovery values for the medical-surgical unit studied. Input variable and output values are explained below.

Output Values

Columns 1 and 4 of the output section represent the quantity (i.e., number of patients for each DRG type treated) in both the base period and the current period, respectively. Columns 2 and 5 are the corresponding average reimbursement rates (price) for each DRG during the base and current periods. Columns 3 and 6 represent the value (given as *quantity x price*, or *column 1 x column 2*). Before explaining the calculations for the input section of Table 6-2, it is helpful to first refer to Table 6-3 where the underlying relationships among the input factors are presented.

Table 6-2. A computational framework for MFPMM application.

	Period 1 (Base Period)			Period 2 (Current Period)			Weighted Change Ratios			Cost/Rev. Ratio		Productivity Ratios		Weighted Performance Ratios			Dollar Effects on Profits		
	Q1	P1	V1	Q2	P2	V2	Q2P1/Q1P1	Q2P2/Q2P1	Q2P2/Q1P1	Period 1 V1/ΣV1	Period 2 V2/ΣV2	Period 1	Period 2	ΔPdy	ΔPR	ΔPfy	ΔPdy	ΔPR	ΔPfy
Column#	1	2	3	4	5	6	7	8	9	10	11	12	13	14	15	16	17	18	19
Outputs:																			
DRG# 127	6	3612	21672	7	3634	25438	1.17	1.01	1.17										
DRG# 096	2	3178	6356	3	3610	10830	1.50	1.14	1.70										
DRG# 089	8	5085	40680	6	4902	29412	0.75	0.96	0.72										
Total Outputs:			68708			65680	0.95	1.01	0.96										
Inputs:																			
Direct Nursing Care	681.6	13.34	9093	840	13.34	11206	1.23	1.00	1.23	0.130	0.171	7.56	5.83	0.77	1.01	0.78	-2546	91	-2455
Indirect Nursing Care	142pd	16.87	2396	175pd	16.87	2952	1.23	1.00	1.23	0.040	0.045	28.68	22.13	0.77	1.01	0.78	-671	24	-647
Room & bed (physical)	142pd	29	4118	175pd	29	5075	1.23	1.00	1.23	0.060	0.077	16.68	12.83	0.77	1.01	0.78	-1153	41	-1112
Variable Overhead	142pd	24.60	3493	175pd	24.6	4305	1.23	1.00	1.23	0.050	0.066	19.67	15.17	0.77	1.01	0.78	-978	35	-943
Fixed Overhead	--	--	2249	--	--	2249	--	--	1.00	0.030	0.034	30.55	29.20	--	--	0.96	--	--	90
Ancillary (weighted average)	16p	1020	16320	16p	1724	27582	1.00	1.69	1.69	0.240	0.420	4.21	4.00	0.95	0.59	0.57	-112	-11802	-11914
Total Inputs:			37669			53369	1.13	1.28	1.44	0.550	0.813	1.82	1.64	0.84	0.79	0.67	-6592	-11489	-18081
Key:	Q1 = Quantity in period 1 Q2 = Quantity in period 2	P1 = Price in period 1 P2 = Price in period 2	V1 = Value (Q1.P1) in period 1		V2 = Value (Q2.P2) in period 2				pd = patient days p = patients	I1 = Input in period 1 I2 = Input in period 2		Pdy = Productivity			PR = Price Recovery		Pfy = Profitability		Δ = change in

Table 6-3. Unit costs (inputs) as a function of variables.

Input factors	Stated as a function of:			
	Patients days	Patient acuity (hours)	Wage dollars	Number of patients
1. Direct nursing care costs	X	X	X	
2. Indirect nursing care costs	X		X	
3. Room and bed (physical) costs	X		X	
4. Variable overhead	X		X	
5. Ancillary care costs			X	X

Input Variables

Columns 7 through 9 represent weighted change ratios. Column 7 shows us the period price and cost weighted change ratios for outputs and inputs. For example, this hospital can draw the following conclusions:

- In period 2, this nursing unit treated 17% more patients of DRG 127.

- Using the weighted change ratio, this nursing unit treated 5% fewer patients in period 2 than period 1, despite the fact that the actual patient counts were the same. The calculation is shown below:

$$\frac{\sum Q_2 P_1}{\sum Q_1 P_1} = \frac{7(3612)+3(3178)+6(5085)}{6(3612)+2(3178)+8(5085)} = 0.95$$

- 23% more direct nursing care was provided in period 2 than in period 1.

$$\frac{Q_2 P_1}{Q_1 P_1} = \frac{840 \times 13.34}{681.6 \times 13.34} = 1.23$$

- 23% more indirect nursing care was provided in period 2 than in period 1.

$$\frac{Q_2 P_1}{Q_1 P_1} = \frac{175 \times 16.87}{142 \times 16.87} = 1.23$$

- Similarly, room and bed and variable overhead inputs, each went up by 23% in period 2.

- Ancillary resource consumption did not change from period 1 to period 2.

$$\frac{Q_2 P_1}{Q_1 P_1} = \frac{16 \times 1020}{16 \times 1020} = 1.0$$

- 13% more input resources were consumed in period 2 than in period 1. The total price-weighted and indexed change in inputs consumed is given as follows:

$$\frac{840(13.34) + 175(16.87) + 175(29) + 175(24.60) + 16(1020)}{681.6(13.34) + 142(16.87) + 142(29) + 142(24.60) + 16(1020)}$$

$$= \frac{39,858}{35,419} = 1.13$$

Column 8 gives the change in unit prices and unit costs from period 1 to period 2 with no change in quality. The following conclusions can be made:

- For DRG 127, for example, the unit price went up by 1% in period 2 as shown below:

$$\frac{Q_2 P_2}{Q_2 P_1} = \frac{7(3634)}{7(3612)} = 1.01$$

- For all three DRGs, prices went up by 1% in period 2. That is,

$$\frac{\sum Q_2 P_2}{\sum Q_2 P_1} = \frac{65680}{65328} = 1.01$$

• Direct nursing care wages and salaries, as well as input prices, stayed the same between periods 1 and 2. However, ancillary costs increased by 69% in period 2.

• Input resources cost 28% more in period 2 than in period 1 as shown below:

$$\frac{840(13.34)+175(16.87)+175(24.60)+16(1724)}{840(13.34)+175(16.87)+175(29)+175(24.60)+16(1020)}$$

$$=\frac{51,122}{39,858}=1.28$$

Column 9 represents the simultaneous effect of price/costs and quantities. The following observations can be made:

• Revenues increased by 17% in period 2 for DRG 127 and by 70% for DRG 096. Revenues, however, decreased by 28% for DRG 089 in period 2. The calculation for DRG 127 is shown below:

$$\frac{Q_2 P_2}{Q_1 P_1}=\frac{7(3634)}{6(3612)}=1.17$$

• The output rows in Column 9 show that this hospital's nursing unit had a 4% decrease in revenues (for the three DRGs) in period 2 as follows:

$$\frac{\sum Q_2 P_2}{\sum Q_1 P_1}=\frac{65,680}{68,708}=0.96$$

• The input rows in column 9 show increases in costs from period 1 to period 2. Direct nursing care costs increased by 23% and ancillary cost increased by 69%.

$$\frac{Q_2 P_2}{Q_1 P_1}=\frac{840(13.34)}{681.6(13.34)}=1.23$$

• For the three DRGs examined, total input (costs) increased by 44% from period 1 to period 2 as shown below:

$$\frac{\sum Q_2 P_2}{\sum Q_1 P_1} = \frac{51,122}{35,419} = 1.44$$

Note, however, that revenues decreased by 4% during the same period for the three DRGs as shown in the output value of column 9.

Columns 10 and 11 depict cost/revenue ratios and help to focus attention on the major cost drivers. For example, direct nursing care cost was 13% of the total revenues in the base period and 17.1% in the current period. Ancillary costs on the other hand, were 24% of the total revenue in the base period, and 42% in the current period. The equation for determining the percentage of direct nursing care costs of total revenue is as follows:

$$9093/68,708 = 0.13$$

Columns 12 and 13 are the absolute productivity ratios for periods 1 and 2, respectively. In a sense, these are partial productivity ratios (given as the ratio of output to one class of input). For example, direct labor (direct nursing care) productivity in period 1 is 7.56, which is derived as follows:

$$68,708/9093 = 7.56$$

The partial productivity for direct nursing care in period 2 is given as 5.83. Note that the combined productivity for the three DRGs examined is given as 1.82 in period 1 and 1.64 in period 2 (column 13). One of the advantages of partial productivity measures is that they can be used for monitoring changes in resource consumption with respect to changes in output.

Columns 14 through 16 represent the weighted performance indexes. Column 14 gives us the rate of change of productivity from period 1 to period 2. The following inferences can be made from these columns:

• For direct nursing care, the productivity index is 0.77 (0.95/ 1.23). Therefore, partial productivity due to direct nursing care is down 23%. The same conclusions can be made about indirect nursing costs, room and bed (physical) costs, and variable overhead costs. Ancillary costs experienced only a 5% decrease. Overall, productivity is down 16%.

• Column 15 gives the rate of change of price-recovery or prices over costs from period 1 to period 2. It can be seen that price recovery is up 1% in four of the six input variables. However, price recovery is down 41% for ancillary and 21% for all inputs. The sample calculation for direct nursing care is given as

$$1.01/1.00 = 1.01 \text{ (from column 8)}$$

In the case of ancillary costs, the inference is that suppliers increased their costs to the hospital faster than it raised its prices to its patients. Some of the changes are minimal because the hospital does not control prices in a DRG environment.

• Column 16 depicts the simultaneous change in prices/costs and the quantities consumed. According to this index, direct nursing care contributed to a 22% decrease in profitability from period 1 to period 2. Overall, profits decreased by 33% due to the slight decline in productivity and price recovery. The 22% figure for direct nursing costs is derived as follows:

$$0.96/1.23 = 0.78$$

Columns 17 through 19 depict the dollar effect on profit changes from period 1 to period 2 for productivity and price recovery. For example, price recovery for ancillary was a loss of $11,802 contributing to 65% of the overall loss of profits of $18,081. In the bottom line analysis, the nursing unit and hospital became $18,081 less profitable from period 1 to period 2. In column 19 for example, it is shown that direct nursing care drained profits by $2,455.

CONCLUSIONS

While the primary objective of health-care organizations is to provide quality health care to patients, the need for efficiency in the use of resources is increasingly making this objective difficult to manage. The Multi-Factor Productivity Measurement Model provides a powerful method for monitoring the economic health of health-care organizations. The model successfully links productivity and profitability in a dynamic process.

The simplicity of the model makes it easy for both nursing and hospital administrators to use and understand. Perhaps the most important feature of the model is its ability to help a hospital identify its major cost drivers. Once identified, a hospital can begin to develop plans for controlling these costs.

One limitation of this model, however, is in the types and volume of information needed to use it. A precise and computer-based information management system is critical to the success of this model. A hospital that still relies on a file-based system will have some difficulty in implementing the MFPMM. Also, such a computerized record-keeping system will make it easy to perform this analysis on all 490 DRGs for various nursing units. Also, for non DRG reimbursement such as per diem, percent change, or indigent care, the model becomes increasingly more complicated.

EXERCISES

6-1. Using the top ten DRGs (in terms of length of stay), perform an analysis using the procedure described in the chapter. How do your results compare to the results reported in the case example?

6-2. What are some of the limitations of the MFPMM? Discuss how you might overcome the limitations.

6-3. Discuss how your organization might use the concept of price recovery to achieve better economic efficiency.

BIBLIOGRAPHY

American Hospital Association (AHA). 1986. *Hospital Departmental Profiles, Second edition.* Alan J. Goldberg and Robert A. DeNoble, editors. Applied Management Systems, Inc.

Anderson, M. L. 1980. Productivity monitoring: A key element of productivity. *Cost Containment in Hospitals.* Efraim Turban, editor. Rockville, MD: Aspen Systems Corporation.

Arndt, M. and B. Skydell. 1982. Inpatient nursing services: Productivity and cost. *Costing Out Nursing Services: Pricing Our Product.* National League for Nursing. Pub. no. P.135.

Benson, G. C. 1981. A model to measure the productivity of nursing personnel in acute care hospitals. *Spring Annual Conference and World Productivity Congress Proceedings.* Norcross, GA: Institute of Industrial Engineers. p. 230.

Bertz, Edward J. 1983. Hospital productivity plays key role under prospective pricing. *The Hospital Manager.* Chicago, IL: American Hospital Association. November-December.

Curtin, L. L. and C. Zurlage. 1986. Nursing productivity: From data to definition. *Nursing Management.* 17(6):32.

Dennis, L. C. and R. Jelinek. 1976. A review and evaluation of nursing productivity. *Health Manpower References.* DHEW Pub. no. (HRA) 77-15.

Dennis, L. C., M. Dunn, and G. Benson. 1980. An empirical model for measuring nursing productivity in acute care hospitals.

DiVestea, Nancy. 1984. The challenging health-care system: An overview. *DRGs: Changes and Challenges.* Franklin A. Shaffer, ed. New York: National League for Nursing. Pub. no. 20-1959.

Edwardson, S. R. 1985. Measuring nursing productivity. *Nursing Economics.* 3(1):9-14.

Giovannetti, P. 1986. A report on the national invitational conference on nursing productivity. Georgetown University. October, p. 41.

Gray, S. P. and W. Steffy. 1983. *Hospital Cost Containment Through Productivity Management*. New York: Van Nostrand Reinhold Company.

Jelinek, R. C. and D. Lyman. 1976. A review and evaluation of nursing productivity. Bethesda, MD. DHEW Pub. no. (HRA) 77-15.

Levine, Eugene. 1984. Some issues in nursing productivity. *Costing Out Nursing: Pricing Our Product*. Franklin A. Shaffer, ed. New York: National League for Nursing. Pub. no. 20-1982. p. 237.

Levey, S. and N. Loomba. 1973. *Health Care Administration: A Managerial Perspective*. Philadelphia: J. B. Lippincott.

Maraldo, P. J. 1984. The challenge: Health care in crisis. *DRGs: Changes and Challenges*. Franklin A. Shaffer, ed. New York: National League for Nursing. Pub. no. 20-1959

Meyer, D. 1985. Costing nursing care with the GRASP system. *Costing Out Nursing: Pricing Our Product*. Franklin A. Shaffer, ed. New York: National League for Nursing. Pub. no. 20-1982.

Mitchell, M., J. Miller, J. Welches, and D. Walker. 1984. Determining cost of direct nursing care by DRGs. *Nursing Management*. 15(4).

Mundel, M. E. 1976. Measures of productivity. *Industrial Engineering*. Norcross, GA: Institute of Industrial Engineers. 8(5):24-26.

Nunamaker, T. R. Measuring routine nursing service efficiency: a comparison of cost per patient day and data development analysis models. *Health Services Research*. 18(2). Part I.

Omachonu, V. K. and R. Nanda.1988. A conceptual framework for hospital nursing unit productivity measurement. *Industrial Engineering*. Norcross, GA: Institute of Industrial Engineers. 20(5).

_____. 1988. Developing a new data base for hospital productivity information management. *Proceedings of the 10th Annual Computers and Industrial Engineering Conference*. Dallas, TX.

_____. 1989. Measuring productivity: outcome vs. output. *Nursing Management*. 20(4).

Riley, W. J. and V. Schefers. 1984. Nursing operations as a profit center. *Nursing Management*. 15(4):43.

_____. 1983. Costing nursing services. *Nursing Management*. 14:40-43.

Shaffer, F. 1984. *DRGs: Changes and Challenges*. New York: National League for Nursing. Pub. no. 20-1959.

Sink, D. S. 1985. *Productivity Management: Planning, Measurement and Evaluation, Control and Improvement*. New York, NY: John Wiley & Sons.

Sumanth, D. J. 1984. *Productivity Engineering and Management*. New York, NY: McGraw-Hill Book Company.

Walker, D. 1983. The cost of nursing in hospitals. *Journal of Nursing Administration*. 13:13-18.

7 Productivity Improvement In Health-Care Organizations

Health-care administrators are constantly searching for techniques that will increase revenues, save costs, improve quality, and use resources efficiently. The successful deployment of such techniques must be preceded by a clear understanding of how changes to output, input, and quality can cause the desired result. It is becoming increasingly challenging for hospitals to operate in an economically restrained environment. Costs and profitability have become critical issues in the continued survival of hospitals. These issues are especially pressing today, owing to the pressures imposed by the introduction of DRGs and the prospective payment system. The need for a formalized approach for maintaining economy and competitiveness is growing. Today's health-care environment calls for a complete knowledge of costs and quality, and what techniques can be used to effect them.

TOTAL PRODUCTIVITY ON THE BASIS OF INDIVIDUAL DIAGNOSIS

Diagnosis-based productivity is defined as the ratio of diagnosis-based output to input. Diagnosis-based output is stated in terms of the total DRG revenues generated by patients treated for a given diagnosis during the productivity measurement period. Input is the cost of the resources consumed in treating patients of the specific DRG. Some inputs cannot be entirely traced to a given DRG, therefore, such inputs are adjusted by a factor which is given as the ratio of total patient days in that DRG to the overall patient days (all patients) in the unit. Both input and output are adjusted to base period prices. From these definitions, the total productivity (for a unit or diagnosis) can be stated generally as follows:

$$\text{Total Productivity} = \frac{\text{Output (O)}}{\text{Input (I)}} \times \text{QualityFactor(Q)}$$

I = Input (stated in terms of resources consumed)
O = Output (stated in terms of DRG revenues generated)
Q = Quality factor (stated in terms of computed score generated from a valid quality assurance survey instrument)

Note: Input and output are adjusted to base period prices.

Table 7-1 presents nine possible scenarios for productivity increases. It is by no means an exhaustive list of all possible scenarios for productivity increases, but is a starting point for understanding the complex interrelationships among all three parameters of productivity. The nine scenarios can be classified into the following three basic strategies for productivity improvement:

Quality-based strategies. If hospitals are to attain a competitive edge in the health-care market, they must pursue a policy of continuous improvement in the quality of care they provide. Scenarios that emphasize an increase in the level of quality of care (over a previous period), such as scenarios 5, 6, 7, 8, and 9, have to be considered the premium techniques.

Input/output strategies. Scenarios that emphasize changes in output and input with no change in quality score are referred to

Table 7-1. Table of attributes and parameters.

Attributes		+M	-M	+H	-H	0
Parameters						
Scenario #1	I	S				
	O			S		
	Q					S
Scenario #2	I					S
	O		S			
	Q					S
Scenario #3	I		S			
	O					S
	Q					S
Scenario #4	I				S	
	O		S			
	Q					S
Scenario #5	I		S			
	O					S
	Q	S				
Scenario #6	I					S
	O					S
	Q	S				
Scenario #7	I		S			
	O	S				
	Q	S				
Scenario #8	I	S				
	O	S				
	Q			S		
Scenario #9	I	S		S		
	O					
	Q	S				

+M: Signifies a moderate increase in I, O, or Q over the previous period.

-M: Signifies a moderate decrease in I, O, or Q over the previous period.

+H: Signifies a higher rate of increase in any one of I, O or Q, when compared to one or both of the remaining I, O, or Q parameter(s). For example, if the output increased from a previous period level of 4 to the present period level of 10, while input also increased from 2 to 4 during the same period, then although output and input have both increased, output increased at a higher rate.

-H: Signifies a higher rate of decrease in any one of I, O, or Q, when compared to one or both of the remaining I, O, or Q parameter(s).

O: Signifies the parameters I, O, or Q remained unchanged when compared to the previous period.

as input/output strategies. Those cases are illustrated by scenarios 1 and 4. They represent short-term strategies that may be implemented in order to control the efficient use of resources. If such strategies are to be used, acceptable levels of quality must first be ensured.

Pure strategies. Scenarios that reflect a variance in either input or output while keeping the remaining input or output score and the quality score unchanged are referred to as pure strategies. Pure strategies are depicted by scenarios 2 and 3. Scenario 2 shows unchanged levels of Q or I, while varying O; scenario 3 shows unchanged levels of Q and O, while varying I.

It should be pointed out that quality-based strategies are preferable because they directly affect the customer. The other strategies are short-term strategies.

PRODUCTIVITY IMPROVEMENT TECHNIQUES

The techniques presented below are referred to as productivity improvement techniques only because they can directly or indirectly affect the productivity equation presented earlier in this chapter. They are strategies that will affect input, output, and quality. These techniques should be used with a quality improvement program, otherwise they may not move an organization toward the needs of its customers. Each strategy must be managed efficiently in order to realize the full benefits of productivity improvement.

Market Promotion and Advertising

Advertising and promotion have traditionally been used to increase sales in both service and manufacturing industries. Prior to the introduction of the prospective payment system, advertising and promotion in hospitals received limited consideration. With increasing competition among hospitals and a growing desire on the part of the buyer of health care to shop around for good service, hospitals are turning to advertising and promotion tactics. According to Steiber (1988), hospital advertising totaled $786 million in 1987, a 45 percent increase over 1986 figures. The average hospital spent an estimated

$158,300 per year on advertising. When salary estimates and other marketing costs are added into the advertising budgets, that number increases to $294,237. Print advertising continues to be the preferred mode of advertising in health care and accounts for approximately 50 percent of advertising costs. The largest portion of that expenditure is spent on daily newspaper insertions.

The success of an advertising campaign depends, to a large extent, on the message it seeks to convey and the manner in which the message is conveyed. Advertising messages that highlight the special features and strengths of a hospital tend to be more effective than very general ones. According to a survey conducted by HealthSell Inc., the practice of employing a full-time sales person in hospitals is common (*AHA News*, December 19, 1988). More than 75 percent of the respondents stated that at least one person whose primary responsibility is to sell a service or a product is employed by their hospitals.

Contract Management Programs

Hospital administrators are searching for more economical and viable means of providing quality patient care. The management of functions—from outpatient surgery and treatment of cancer patients to bill collection—is increasingly being performed on a contractual basis by firms specializing in health-care management.

About 88 percent of nearly 400 hospitals surveyed in 1989 by American Hospital Publishing, Inc. in conjunction with HPI Health Care Services, Inc., are using contract management in their hospitals. The survey reveals that contract management is being used by:

- 38 percent of hospitals for laundry services
- 30 percent for physical therapy
- 29 percent for food services
- 26 percent for emergency services
- 21 percent for housekeeping
- 15 percent for pharmacy
- 10 percent for respiratory therapy

Other areas in which contract management can be applied include coma care centers, cancer centers, ambulatory care centers, and financial services. Now, although quality remains a vital part of contract management services, cost issues are taking on greater significance. Outside contractors can, and do, save money for their clients through economies of scale. It should be pointed out that, although contract management has its appeal, it is not for every hospital. Its cost/benefits should be thoroughly investigated.

Specialist/Generalist Practitioners

The increasing shortage of nurses forces hospital administrators to make tough choices between specialty and generalist nurses. For example, if a given nursing unit experiences abnormally high increases in coronaries in winter, but relatively few the rest of the year, perhaps the unit would do better by contracting with a cardiac clinician full-time for four months during the winter rather than paying a full-time yearly salary for someone who may be underutilized during the summer months. This would result in tremendous savings in direct nursing care cost. On the other hand, it is reported that of the top ten physician specialists, cardiologists brought hospitals the most inpatient revenue in 1987, and cardiovascular surgeons accounted for the most revenues per patient (Carlsen 1988).

Specialized Units/Patients Grouping

Input reduction can be achieved by grouping patients into specialized units. For high-volume DRGs, a specialized unit could enhance the consolidation of resources. For example, grouping patients with routine three- to four-day surgeries into a short-stay surgical unit allows for more efficient staffing and ultimately reduced operating costs. When such patients are scattered throughout the hospital, it is difficult to manage that category of demand.

Increasing Physicians' Cost Consciousness

As much as 80 percent of the expenditures for medical care are for services prescribed by physicians, despite the fact that physicians' fees represent only about 20 percent of health-care costs. Physicians drive almost every aspect of the demand for health care; the physician makes the decision whether to admit a patient, determines if and when surgery is necessary, determines the types and number of tests to be performed, determines what types of drugs to prescribe, and has the final say over the length of hospitalization. Many studies suggest that when doctors become more aware of the costs of the resources which their patients consume, they tend to prescribe more efficiently. The ability to make cost information available (for all resources) to physicians on a regular basis is paramount to the success of this program.

Constant Quality Improvement Programs

If a hospital is to gain a competitive edge through the quality of the services it provides, then the activity of quality improvement must be a continuous process. Involvement at all levels of the organization is necessary for the program's success. It is significant to note that while full participation is necessary for the success of any quality improvement program, the leadership and participation of nursing is critical. Nurses come in contact with the patients on a daily basis and almost all of the hands-on care delivery is provided by nurses. However, each participant in the care delivery process (doctors, nurses, radiologists, pharmacists, etc.) must carefully formulate goals with respect to quality assurance, and work together toward the joint accomplishment of such goals. The effort must be never-ending.

Management Engineering Cost Reduction Process

A management engineering cost reduction process involves the application of traditional management engineering and operations research (time and motion study, work sampling, facility design and layout, simulation, mathematical programming, scheduling, staffing, capacity planning, product mix and management, etc.) to achieve system efficiency. Today's health-care environment requires that the pursuit of such cost reduction processes be balanced with the need for adequate quality of care delivery. The role of management engineering must be patient-centered.

Improved Information System Management

As a general rule, the primary objective of an information management system should be to provide the right type and amount of information to the right place, at the right time. This includes information provided to patients, medical records, radiology, pharmacy, financial and accounting services, nursing units, etc. For years now, management engineers have documented the fact that nurses spend 40 to 60 percent of their time on paper work. The concept of bedside terminals has been utilized successfully in many hospitals to address this problem. The greatest benefit of bedside terminals lies in the ability to free nurses from the tremendous paper shuffle, and give them more time for hands-on nursing care. A good information management system must capture and present total resource consumption information by DRG, by day, and by nursing unit.

Hospitality Management Program

Quality assurance is not a departmental activity; it is the essence of health-care practice. Patients do not just buy health care; they buy expectations. Patients expect to get well, be treated promptly, courteously, and in the right manner. Patients also expect that the doctors, nurses, and other personnel will do all the right things from a conformance-to-standards point of view.

Quality of care has become the primary yardstick by which health-care organizations are judged. Hospitality considerations and other aspects of care that influence the customer's perception can no longer be ignored. Hospitals that go out of their way to encourage complaints and remedy them reap significant rewards. A massive education, training, and nursing hospitality management campaign is critical if a hospital desires to attract more "buyers" to its health-care delivery facility.

Employee Recognition and Motivation Programs

In most cases, such programs begin with a suggestion box system or a quality improvement idea contest. The importance of such programs lies in their ability to motivate employees to participate in the improvement and growth process of the organization and to adequately recognize employee participation. For a recognition program to be successful, it has to be a formal program and everyone should be aware of its existence. The program should have as its leadership a group of people who are drawn from various departments of the hospital, including the nursing units. The various forms of recognition may include moderate cash awards, special mention in the hospital newsletter or bulletin, photo recognition on the hospital's bulletin board, a monthly name-recognition on the hospital's electronic billboard, or the assignment of a reserved parking space to employees. Another factor critical to the success of employee recognition and motivation programs is emphasizing and recognizing team or group efforts as opposed to only individual contributions.

Adequate Unit/Patient Support Services

In many hospital environments, some of the responsibilities for providing unit and patient support services rests on the shoulders of licensed, professional nurses. As a consequence, the nurse's time is shared between performing those duties that do not require a licensed professional and the duties of actual patient care. Having an adequate nursing unit and patient support services would allow the nursing professional more time to concentrate on providing quality nursing care. In general, an adequate nursing unit and patient support services program uses support staff instead of licensed, professional nurses for transporting patients for admissions, transfers, and discharges; moving patients in and out of bed; counting dressing cards; ordering and restacking unit supplies; collecting patients' trays after meals; transporting equipment; collecting and labeling specimens; maintaining a clean and organized working environment; and charting lab slips into medical records.

Education of Staff

While clinical expertise remains a strong criteria for evaluating the strength of a hospital, the survival of a hospital also depends on the training and education of its staff in areas other than clinical. Training and education in areas such as effective service delivery techniques, business orientation in health care, and quality and customer satisfaction are as important as clinical training. Many hospitals today are sponsoring their nurses and doctors through business degree programs, short courses, and seminars. Quality and productivity can be enhanced through the provision of adequate training and education.

Flexible Staffing

Some positions at the hospital are fixed full- or part-time positions. Others are flexible positions, with a guaranteed minimum number of hours and a larger total number of hours that the employee must work, if asked. In addition, a hospital may have nurses who work on a per diem. This staffing system allows unit administrators to make daily staffing adjustments to match the unit's occupancy. For example, a full-time staff is used for peak demand, while part-time and per diem staff are used for normal demand.

Ancillary Services Cost Containment Programs

Doctors and patients depend immensely on the services provided by hospital ancillary service departments. The responsiveness of these departments to doctors' requirements—measured in terms of range of service, scope of coverage, and speed of response—significantly affects a hospital's quality of care, the length of stay of patients, and occupancy rate. The following is a brief discussion on selected ancillary services, their impact on costs, and techniques that can be employed in each to improve productivity. It is by no means exhaustive, but is an attempt to recognize some of the powerful improvement ideas currently utilized by hospitals.

Radiology services. According to Peterson, et al. (1980), "...of all the ancillary services, those rendered by this [radiology] department have the greatest impact on a hospital's ability to achieve a low length of stay. Turn-around time and hours of availability are critical factors in achieving reduced costs through radiology." Perry and Baum (1976) in their discussion of radiology department performance, state that "delays in handling diagnostic reports contribute directly to increased patient-care costs and the length of stay." They refer, in fact, to a 1971 study by Gertman and Becker in which it was found that, at the time, "approximately sixteen percent of the inappropriate days of hospital stay were caused by delayed radiology reports." A day was defined as "inappropriate" if the major reason for that day's stay was not directly related to patient diagnosis or treatment. Peterson, et al. (1980) gave three reasons why radiological availability and turn-around time have an important impact on a patient's rate of progress.

- Radiological procedures usually constitute key elements of the diagnostic process; therefore, treatment (usually by surgery) and recovery cannot begin until they have been completed. Not diagnosing a patient prior to admission can seriously affect radiology turn around time and patient length of stay.

- The radiology process itself is complex even when the X-ray procedure itself is simple. Therefore, the opportunities for causing significant delays to any or all patients are considerable. Because the process involves a series of steps, the effective management of working and waiting times are critical for cost reduction. The process can include up to eleven steps:

1. Ordering the test by the physicians
2. Scheduling the test
3. Transporting and managing the patient while waiting for an available room
4. Taking the actual X-ray
5. Returning the patient
6. Interpreting the results
7. Typing the report

8. Delivering the report to the nursing station
9. Including the report on the patient's chart
10. Physician's study of the report
11. Physician's consultation with the radiologist (if necessary)

• The availability and working habits of radiologists are critical because they are personally involved in performing special procedures, interpreting X-rays, and consulting with physicians.

Laboratory services. Pathologists and physicians agree that patient progress is related to the availability and speed of service that the laboratory provides. Response time, from a doctor's perspective (the total time that elapses between a physician's order for a test and the availability of the test results to him) is a critical factor in productivity improvement. According to Peterson, et al. (1980), laboratory response time has three components:

1. The hours and days during which laboratory services are available for tests and consultations

2. The length of time that the laboratory requires to perform the test and record the test results

3. The efficiency with which requests and specimens are collected and test results are delivered and placed on patient's charts

   Peterson, et al. (1980) note that an effective way of improving response times is by "advancing blood collection times in the morning to a point where the test results are on the chart by the time most doctors make their morning rounds." Also, for incoming patients without preadmission testing, the following procedures can be put in place to minimize their length of stay:

• collecting blood immediately before patients proceed to their rooms
• establishing a priority system in the laboratory
• establishing flexible and adequate staffing patterns in the

afternoons and evenings (especially for patients admitted in the afternoons)

Preadmission testing (PAT). The length of stay for elective patients can be substantially minimized by completing the diagnostic aspects of a patient's care prior to admission. The critical factors in the success of PAT programs lies in the degree of emphasis placed on the program, the scope of available services, and the frequency with which it is employed. Peterson, et al. (1980) further note the following as keys to a successful PAT program:

- an institutional commitment to provide the necessary staffing and resources for an effective program

- services that are readily available to patients at convenient times and locations

- timely delivery of test results to physicians

- a medical staff that understands the importance of the program (including its potential impact on bed availability) and encourages patients to use it

Operating rooms. More than half of all patients undergo a surgical procedure during the course of their hospitalization, according to Peterson, et al. (1980). It is no surprise, therefore, that the availability of adequate operating time largely affects the flow of patients, the length of their stay, and the occupancy rate of the institution. Also affected is the ability of a surgeon and his elective patient to plan and schedule admission to the hospital. Thus, operating room availability is a convenience and competitiveness factor. The benefits of ample operating room time include the following:

- Patients who have been admitted for diagnosis or for a medical problem that is later found to require surgery are promptly accommodated.

- Fewer surgeries are postponed which results in less disruption of surgeon's and patent's schedules.

- Length of stay is reduced because more surgeries can be scheduled for early in the day.

Hospital pharmacy. There is an increasing need for hospital pharmacists to team up with medical staffs and administration to tackle the growing health-care costs. In a 1990 national survey conducted by the American Society of Hospital Pharmacists (ASHP) (Crawford 1990), it was revealed that pharmacists are making significant progress toward drug use control. For example, 70 percent of the hospitals surveyed had centralized services; 43.5 percent had centralized services with daily visits to patient care areas by pharmacists; and 26.5 percent had centralized services with occasional visits. In the ASHP survey, respondents were asked if there was a computerized pharmacy system in the hospital and, if so, whether the system was used for inpatient or ambulatory-patient services. A computerized pharmacy system was defined as a computer that, at a minimum, maintains patient drug profiles and generates prescription-fill or dispensing lists. The survey results show that 63.9 percent of the respondents had computerized systems in 1990, compared with 52.1 in 1987.

Technology Management

The effective management of technology can have a tremendous impact on productivity and quality. The availability of state-of-the-art technology is among the factors physicians consider when selecting a hospital for their patients. The management of technology involves the continuous activities of prepurchase planning, purchasing, maintenance, and evaluation. Further discussion of the importance of managing technology in a health-care environment can be found in Chapter Ten.

Employee Selection/Training

Selecting appropriate health-care employees is essential for enhancing productivity and quality. For example, some work involved in nursing is a labor of love; not everyone can be a good nurse. Extensive screening is necessary to reduce the probability of hiring a person who loves the salary but not the job. Goals and expectations must be adequately communicated to staff members, and a formal employee development program should be in place if the quality of labor is to be well managed.

Table 7-2 suggests techniques listed above that can be applied to achieve the goals presented in the scenarios at the first of the chapter.

Table 7-2. Relationship between scenarios and improvement techniques.

Scenario Number	Techniques
1	1, 3, 5, 8
2	3, 5, 8
3	2, 3 ,4 , 5, 6, 7, 10, 13, 14
4	2, 3, 4, 5, 6, 7, 10, 13
5	2, 3, 4, 5, 6, 7, 8, 9, 10, 11, 12, 13, 14
6	2, 6, 8, 9, 10, 11, 12, 16
7	1, 2, 3, 4, 5, 6, 7, 8, 9, 10, 11, 12, 13, 14
8	1, 2, 3, 6, 8, 9, 10, 11, 12, 15, 16
9	1, 2, 3, 6, 8, 9, 10, 11, 12, 15, 16

Many approaches to productivity and quality improvement in hospitals have been presented in this chapter. Important to the success of any technique or combination of techniques is continuous commitment to the goal of attaining increased productivity and quality. Successful productivity and quality improvement strategies will yield fewer errors, reduced waste, decreased costs, and repeat business.

EXERCISES

7-1. Which, if any, contract management services does your organization use?

7-2. Discuss the advantages and disadvantages of contract management with respect to your facility.

7-3. Which of the productivity improvement techniques presented in the chapter is currently being used in your organization? What has been the greatest challenge since implementation?

BIBLIOGRAPHY

Bartscht, K. L. and R. Coffey. 1977. Management engineering— A method to improve productivity. *Topics in Health Care Financing.* Aspen Systems Corp.

Carlsen, A. 1988. Survey: Cardiologists garner most income for hospitals. *Health Week.* 2(20): 14.

Covert, R. P. and E. G. McNulty. 1981. Management engineering for hospitals. American Hospital Association Publication. pp. 4-10.

Crawford, S. Y. 1990. ASHP national survey of hospital-based pharmaceutical services—1990. *American Journal of Hospital Pharmacy.* December. 47: 2665.

DiVestea, N. 1984. The changing health care system: An overview. *DRGs: Changes and Challenges.* Franklin A. Schaffer, ed. New York: National League for Nursing. Pub. no. 20-1959.

Nanda, R. 1986. Redesigning work systems—a new role for IE. *Fall Industrial Engineering Conference Proceedings.* Norcross, GA: Institute of Industrial Engineers. pp. 222-229.

Omachonu, V. K. and M. Beruvides. 1989. Improving hospital productivity: Patient-unit and hospital-based measures. *International Industrial Engineering Conference Proceedings.* Norcross, GA: Institute of Industrial Engineers.

Omachonu, V. K. and R. Nanda. 1988. IEs in health care management must emphasize client-centered projects which can contain cost while supporting quality. *Industrial Engineering.* Norcross, GA: Institute of Industrial Engineers. 20(10): 66.

_____. 1988. A conceptual framework for hospital nursing unit productivity measurement. *Industrial Engineering.* Norcross, GA: Institute of Industrial Engineers. 20(5):56.

_____. 1988. A diagnosis-based approach to hospital nursing unit productivity measurement. *Proceedings of the Ninth Annual Conference.* Knoxville, TN: American Society for Engineering Management. p. 251.

_____. 1988. Hospital information and technology management under the pricing system. *Technology Management I.* Khalil, et al., eds. Switzerland: Inderscience Enterprises, Ltd. p. 515.

_____. 1988. Developing a new data base for hospital productivity information management. *Proceedings of the Tenth Annual Computers and Industrial Engineering Conference.* Dallas, TX. 15: 277.

_____. 1989. Measuring hospital nursing unit productivity under the new reimbursement scheme. *Productivity Management Frontiers II.* Sumanth, et al., eds. Switzerland: Inderscience Enterprises Ltd. p. 63.

Perry, R. F. and R. F. Baum. 1976. Resource allocation and scheduling for a radiology department. *Cost Control in Hospitals.* John R. Griffith, et al., eds. Ann Arbor, MI: Health Administration Press.

Peterson, J., D. Manchester, and A.Toan. 1980. *Enhancing Hospital Efficiency.* AUPHA Press.

Smalley, H. E. 1982. *Hospital Management Engineering.* Englewood Cliffs, NJ: Prentice-Hall International Series in Industrial and Systems Engineering.

Steiber, S. 1988. Hospital advertising budget grows by 45%. *Hospitals.* 62(6).

8 Physician Practice Patterns and Hospital Efficiency

The participation of physicians in managing and controlling health-care resource consumption is critical to a hospital's survival, both short-term and long-term. According to Gibson, Waldo and Levit (1983) and Wilensky and Rossiter (1983), as much as 80 percent of medical care expenditures are for services prescribed by physicians despite the fact that physicians' fees represent only about 20 percent of health-care costs. Physicians drive almost every aspect of the demand for health care; the physician decides whether to admit a patient, determines the types of tests necessary, determines if and when surgery is necessary, prescribes the types of drugs needed and has the final say over the length of hospitalization. This factor is largely responsible for difficulty in forecasting the demand for hospital services, medical resource consumption, as well as the decline in hospital profit per discharge. Eisenberg (1986) makes the analogy, "like the player-manager of an athletic team, the physician is responsible for calling the plays in medical care as well as working with the others to carry them out." The sphere of physician influence is illustrated in Figure 8-1. A comparison of the degree of control over resource consumption among nurs-

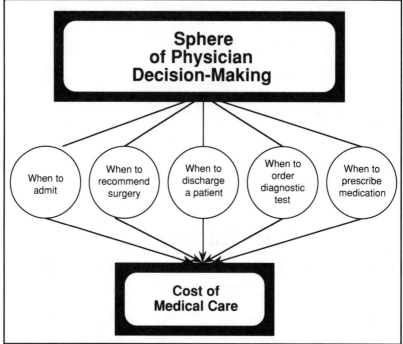

Figure 8-1. Sphere of physician influence on costs.

ing administrators, hospital administrators and medical doctors is illustrated in Figure 8-2. It can be seen from this illustration that, overall, physicians hold the highest degree of control over resource consumption in each category.

One of the most important contributors to the rise in health-care costs has been the expansion in the types and volume of clinical tests performed in laboratories. This point has been made by many researchers over the years. In fact, clinical laboratory testing accounts for approximately 25 percent of hospital charges (Fineberg 1979), and between 1970 and 1975, the average annual increase in the number of laboratory tests was 13.8 percent in hospital laboratories and 15.6 percent in independent non-hospital laboratories (Mohr 1971, Zurke 1976).

VARIATIONS IN PRACTICE PATTERNS

It is generally known that physicians do not all practice alike. For the same diagnosis, one doctor might see the need for

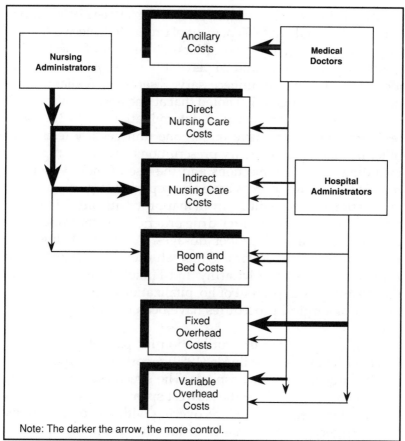

Figure 8-2. Degree of control over resource consumption.

surgery, while another might prefer medical therapy; one physician might elect for a patient to undergo elaborate diagnostic testing, while another physician might elect for a brief period of observation; one doctor might recommend a vaccination, while another doctor might prefer oral medication. These variations lie in the fact that physicians do not have hard and fast rules for determining the volume and types of resources needed by patients.

Bunker (1985) suggests that variation in physicians' practice styles is one cause of inefficiency in medical care. High and unnecessary resource consumption are frequently mentioned when discussing the practice patterns of physicians.

According to Schroeder, Myers, and McPhee (1984), at one teaching hospital, up to 65 percent of orders for selected laboratory tests, 30 percent of stat orders, 11 percent of chest radiographic examinations, and 26 percent of nursing services were judged to be clinically unnecessary. Eisenberg, Williams, Garner, Viale and Smits (1977) noted that at one hospital, about half of patients who had repeated determinations with the same tests were judged to have undergone unnecessary testing. In other instances, unnecessary prescriptions have been reported, including excessive injections and the use of more expensive brands. Literature sources have also reported large numbers of medication errors resulting from inappropriate physician practices, such as illegibly written drug orders, using improper drug abbreviations, and improper dosages. As a result, hospitals waste millions of dollars. Other studies by Gertman and Rustuccia (1981) and McCarthy and Finkel (1978) determined that as much as 25 percent of hospitalization days and about 20 percent of surgical procedures have been considered inappropriate.

In a study on resource utilization for patients undergoing gall bladder operations, Burda (1989) reported on surgery times for 28 surgeons at four hospitals. The speediest surgeon typically spent 21.8 minutes; the slowest spent 84.3 minutes. Their patients fared equally well, recovering without complications. Since surgery can be a matter of life and death, much care is needed to do it right. However, time savings can be realized from eliminating delays and standardizing routine support activities such as pre-surgery preparations.

IMPACT OF PHYSICIAN CHARACTERISTICS

Literature sources suggest that more specialized physicians provide more intensive care than generalists. It is reported by Childs and Hunter (1972), Noren, Frazier, Altman, and DeLozier (1980), and Ernst (1976), that general practitioners (but not necessarily those who are family physicians) order fewer diagnostic tests than do internists. Also, Fishbane and Starfield (1981) noted that pediatricians order significantly more diagnostic tests for common childhood illnesses than general practitioners do.

In general, younger physicians tend to prescribe more services than older ones, according to Childs and Hunter (1972), Eisenberg and Nicklin (1981), Pineault (1977), and Freeborn, Baer, Greenlick, and Bailey (1972). An explanation for this variance may be that older physicians were trained at a time when technology did not play the role in patient care that it does today. These physicians may not have become as accustomed to using diagnostic technology as have their younger colleagues. Alternatively, older physicians have gained clinical experience through years of practice and may not require extensive diagnostic testing to evaluate their patients' needs. Figure 8-3 shows how physician characteristics impact the cost of medical care.

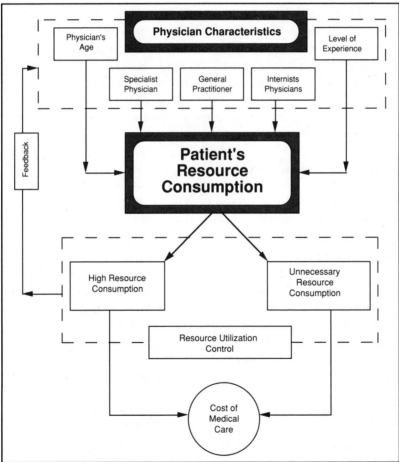

Figure 8-3. Physician characteristics and the cost of medical care.

Misinterpretation of test results is another factor contributing to increased test use, further complicating the goal of determining optimal levels of laboratory testing. An abnormal (positive) test value may lead to further testing in order to verify and explain the result, especially if the test's specificity is low (Grossman 1983). Difficulty in understanding test results is further exacerbated by the sheer growth in the number of different tests now available to physicians. In 1950, there were less than 100 laboratory tests available to the clinician, whereas in 1976, more than 600 laboratory tests were available (Brownfield 1976).

PERSPECTIVES ON COST CONTROL

The role of physicians is critical to the success of any health-care cost containment program. Effectively managing physicians' practice patterns is perhaps the single most important element of hospital cost containment. Various techniques have been suggested for managing this component of cost control, but researchers disagree about the success of such programs. The following is a discussion of some of the techniques for controlling physician-based costs.

Monitoring Practice Style

In view of the status of physicians in hospitals, the biggest question regarding the monitoring of practice style is "who should do the monitoring?" In every hospital, certain physicians seem to be particularly influential in determining group norms of practice style. Such physicians, because of their status and domain of influence, could play the role of educators in the practice of medicine. It is not necessary for such physicians to hold high offices in the hospital; however, they should be regarded highly by their colleagues.

It is often true that doctors who are administratively influential may not be professionally or clinically influential. Clinical leadership has been reported as a strong influence in setting surgical practice patterns by Wennberg and Gittelsohn (1982), and Flood, Scott, Ewy, and Forrest, Jr. (1982). Also, such influence is reported in hospitalization rates and length of stay by Rhee, Luke, and Culverwell (1980), and in the use of diagnostic tests by Freeborn, Baer, Greenlick, and Bailey (1972). Other researchers have also reported the effect of clinically influential physicians in the area of drug prescriptions.

Choosing a group of physicians for monitoring and influencing practice style must transcend the politics of the institution. Regular feedback about how their behavior affects health-care costs must be provided to all participating physicians if the program is to succeed. Feedback provides the physicians the opportunity to regulate their practice patterns. Many successful programs relying on feedback to change physicians' practices have suggested that this approach can improve the quality of care and reduce its cost. If possible, such feedback should be computerized and followed by a face-to-face meeting with a respected member of the medical staff. Faculty physicians are usually suitable for such roles.

Costs Education

Until physicians become more aware of the costs of health-care services and resources, hospitals will realize little success in their cost containment programs. Physicians must become aware of the price of medical care services. Researchers suggest that the price a patient pays for services affects the physicians' patterns of prescribing services (Eisenberg and Williams 1981; Long, Cummings, and Frisof 1983; Hoey, Eisenberg, Spitzer, and Thomas 1982; and Cohen, Jones, Littenberg and Neuhauser 1982). Physicians also seem to be influenced by cost in terms of the number of tests they prescribe. Hoey, Eisenberg, Spitzer, and Thomas (1982) showed that 24 to 38 percent of test ordering is influenced by the price of diagnostic tests depending upon the physician's level of experience.

According to Eisenberg (1986), the following two key challenges face the medical care field:

• convincing clinicians with unusual practice styles to adhere to more commonly accepted practice patterns

• changing the practice styles of physicians whose style of practice may be typical of their colleagues, but who may deviate from an optimal pattern as defined by expert opinions or scientific evidence

In some hospitals today, cost data for resource consumption are printed out on 3" x 5" booklets or cards for physicians to carry for quick and easy reference. Such information can also be supplied by computer to the physician. In a DRG environment, such cost factors need to be matched against the revenues generated by the hospital in order to asses profitability and price recovery. In addition to DRG revenues and cost information, prescribed and actual length of stay information should be made available to physicians on a regular basis. Informal guidelines for the use of health-care resources can sometimes be developed by examining resource use patterns of certain highly respected physicians. Depending on a hospital's organizational structure, these cost improvement information and analysis data can be gathered by the management engineering group.

To educate physicians on the reasons for change, hospitals must share financial and utilization information with physicians. It is widely believed that many health-care administrators are afraid to be tough on physicians for fear that the physicians might take their business elsewhere. The process of change cannot be dictatorial; it should be participative. Physicians may respond more favorably to change if the help of other highly respected physicians is used to elicit their cooperation.

Professional Communication Programs

Effective communication is important for the success of any physician-based cost containment program. Three key factors in communicating needed changes in physicians' practice patterns include:

The source of communication. Who is saying it? How influential is the source? How believable or respectable is the source? Educationally and clinically influential physicians are effective for bringing about change in practice patterns. Usually those physicians to whom others turn for advice are more suitable for this role. Such physicians can also provide informal education and leadership.

The medium of communication. The most effective means of communicating this information is verbally and in person. Communication by mail, memos, newsletters, and so forth are not suitable for this type of program. Recommendations are usually more readily accepted when they are delivered personally by a respected source.

The message itself. The message must be convincing, powerful and to the point. It should be reinforced frequently. Handouts on research studies, cost information, and other visual aids should be used to reinforce the effectiveness of the message. Figure 8-4 shows the information synthesis necessary to support a physician-oriented cost containment program.

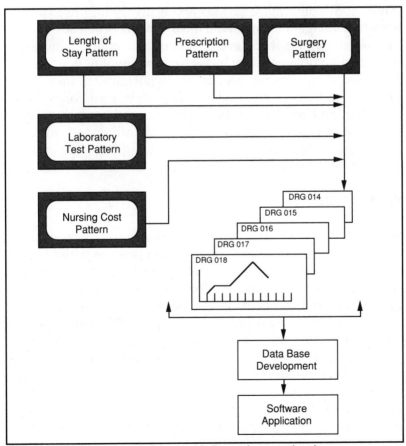

Figure 8-4. Structure of data and information synthesis.

Participation

To achieve effective change in physician practice patterns, physicians must be involved in decisions regarding resource allocation and consumption. In the past, hospitals have operated under two separate power structures—the hospital administrators and the physicians. This separation of the hospital power structure into two (sometimes antagonistic) pillars of influence can have disastrous consequences. It is simply impractical to speak of cost containment efforts without the participation and support of physicians. Pineault (1976) reported that when HMO physicians are involved in administrative roles related to cost containment, reduced use of diagnostic testing is found.

The introduction of DRGs has compelled hospital administrators to become more serious about involving physicians in hospital management, even if it means that hospital administrators must relinquish a certain amount of control. Increased physician involvement can be realized by involving physicians on hospital governing boards, in major capital investment projects, and in short-term and long-term goal formulation, planning, and implementation. The fear of losing the respect and trust of colleagues may do more to influence a doctor to change his or her practice pattern than would the fear of someone looking over his or her shoulder.

Practice Rules

Although seemingly autocratic, some hospitals have tried using administrative rules to control physician practice patterns. This is usually not the best way to control practice patterns, but it is sometimes inevitable. When, for example, a hospital's pharmacy committee limits drugs or a brand of drugs available (for cost reasons), physicians are forced to prescribe within the new boundaries. Such rules can also be applied to diagnostic tests.

Burda (1989) reports on the steps taken by the 783-bed Abbott Northwestern Hospital to change physician practice patterns. The report discusses "the creation of a hospital-wide project in 1988 to develop practice standards for all medical procedures at the facility." The steps taken to implement the project are summarized below:

1. The hospital's cardiologists and cardiac surgeons, together, defined their "best-case scenarios" for a bypass patient's stay at the hospital. The scenario was made up of 15 components, such as optimum length of time a cardiac patient spends in the operating room and in intensive care.

2. The hospital's vice president of medical affairs determined the hospital-wide average for all 15 components and averages for individual physicians.

3. The hospital's vice president of medical affairs also had the task of breaking the news to physicians whose averages exceeded the norms.

4. Results and comparisons were presented to physicians. Improved cardiac care led to a savings in the hospital's bottom line. For example, physicians learned that they can remove patients from respirators earlier resulting in less patient discomfort and less chance for infection. The hospital saves $1,000 for every 24-hour reduction in the time that patients use respirators.

Liability concerns led to the creation of anesthesia practice standards at Harvard Medical Institutions, comprising a network of ten teaching hospitals, a health maintenance organization, and a diabetes foundation (Burda 1989). Five sets of practice standards for anesthesiologists were developed, including a set of requirements for monitoring anesthetized patients.

Since the use of the practice standards, the number of adverse patient reactions from anesthesia declined. Prior to the use of the standards, malpractice losses attributed to anesthesia claims averaged $54,000 per month at the facilities. Losses per month after the standards averaged $27,000. The success of the anesthesia standards caught the attention of other specialists at these hospitals and triggered obstetricians and gynecologists to implement 21 practice standards.

Although the use of practice standards has worked in certain circumstances, it should be pointed out that the emphasis should be on reducing variations in the process. A more permanent solution can be found in establishing specifications that ensure adequate outcome. The process should be managed to ensure consistency and eliminate variations. Although diseases seldom fall into neat categories, knowledge of variations will make physicians more aware of how outcome can be managed.

Control Charts

As discussed in Chapter Four, control charts can be used to monitor physicians' resource utilization practices. A variety of physician activities, such as the time to perform certain surgeries, the number of tests requested for certain DRGs, the LOS for certain DRGs, etc. can be analyzed using control charts. Upper and lower control limits can be established to monitor resource utilization over a given period of time. When activities fall outside of the control limit, a clinically influential physician should determine the special causes of variation. Figure 8-5 illustrates the use of control charts to monitor resource utilization.

Periodic reviews of control charts by DRG, physician, and cost component should follow the information gathering process. It is not necessary to perform this analysis for every DRG; however, it is essential to analyze the ten percent of DRGs that account for 90 percent of a hospital's revenue (or cost). Periodic reviews are necessary even when the practice patterns remain in control. It is suggested that such reviews be conducted only by clinically influential physicians.

Conclusion. The ideal situation for a health-care facility is for members of the medical staff to want to change their practice patterns. A hospital will be better able to accomplish the change if the physicians are convinced that it is appropriate. Forcing a change in practice patterns is undesirable since it is likely to make physicians defensive and may ultimately have a harmful effect on the relationship between the physician and the hospital administration. Changing the way physicians practice requires hard work. Most of all, it calls for the intervention of a clinically influential physician who also knows a thing or two about how to be diplomatic.

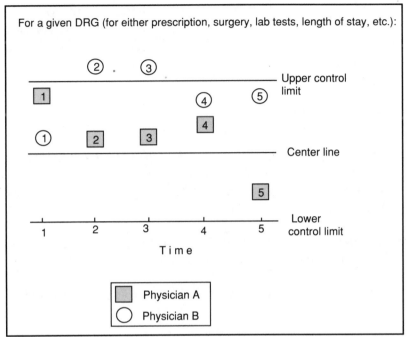

Figure 8-5. Control chart for monitoring resource utilization.

EXERCISES

8-1. Conduct a study to determine if there are any differences between the following categories of physicians in resource utilization (LOS, lab tests, X-ray, EEG. EKG, etc.) for the same patient groups:

- older vs. younger physicians
- specialist vs. non-specialist physicians
- internists vs. non-internists

What conclusions can you draw from your study?

8-2. Does your facility have a formal program for monitoring physicians' practice patterns? If so, is the head of that program an administrator, a clinician, or both? What are the implications of having or not having a clinically influential physician in charge of such a program?

8-3. What percentage of your hospital's expenditures for medical care are for services prescribed by physicians? What is the implication of this figure on the cost of medical care at your facility?

BIBLIOGRAPHY

Brook, R. H., K. Williams, and J. Rolph. 1978. Controlling the use and cost of medical services: The New Mexico experimental medical care review organization—A four-year case study. *Med. Care.* 16 (suppl):1-76.

Brownfield, R. J. and E. Ives. 1976. Creating a data base for the laboratory universe. *Laboratory Management.* 14(22).

Bunker, J. P. 1985. When doctors disagree. *New York Review of Books.* 32(7):8-12.

Burda, D. 1989. Changing physician practice patterns. *Modern Healthcare.* February 17:18.

Childs, A. W. and E. Hunter. 1972. Non-medical factors influencing use of diagnostic x-ray by physicians. *Med. Care.* 10: 323-35.

Cohen, D. I., P. Jones, B. Littenberg, and D. Neuhauser. 1982. Does cost information availability reduce physician test usage? A randomized clinical trial with unexpected findings. *Med. Care.* 20:286-92.

Daniels, M. and S. Schroeder. 1977. Variation among physicians in use of laboratory tests: II. Relation to clinical productivity and outcomes of care. *Med. Care.* 15:482-87.

Eisenberg, J. M. , S. Williams, L. Garner, R.Viale, and H. Smits. 1977. Computer-based audit to detect and correct overutilization of laboratory tests. *Med. Care.* 15:915-921.

Eisenberg, J. M. and S. Williams. 1981. Cost containment and clogging physicians practice behavior: Can the fox learn to guard the chicken coop? *J.A.M.A.* 246:2195-2201.

Eisenberg, J. M. and D. Nicklin. 1981. Use of diagnostic services by physicians in community practice. *Med. Care.* 19:297-309.

Eisenberg, J. M. 1982. The use of ancillary services: A role for utilization review? *Med. Care.* 20:849-861.

_____. 1986. Doctors decisions and the cost of medical care. Health Administration Press Perspectives. Ann Arbor, MI. p. 3.

Ernst, R. 1976. Ancillary production and size of physicians practice. *Inquiry.* 13:371-381.

Fineberg, H. V. 1979. Clinical chemistries: The high cost of low-cost diagnostic tests. *Medical Technology: The Culprit Behind Health Care Costs?* Altman, S. H. and R. Bierdon, eds. DHEW Pub. (PHS) 79-3216.

Fishbane, M. and B. Starfield. 1981. Child health care in the United States: A comparison of pediatricians and general practitioners. *New England Journal of Medicine.* 305:552-556.

Flood, A. B., W. Scott, W. Ewy, and W. Forrest, Jr. 1982. Effectiveness in professional organizations: The impact of surgeons and surgical staff organizations on the quality of care in hospitals. *Health Services Research.* 17:341-366.

Freeborn, D. K., D. Baer, M. Greenlick, and J. Bailey. 1972. Determinants of medical care utilization: Physicians use of laboratory services. *American Journal of Public Health.* 62:846-853.

Gertman, P. M. and J. Rustuccia. 1981. The appropriateness evaluation protocol: A technique for assessing unnecessary days of hospital care. *Med. Care.* 19:855-71.

Gibson, R. M., D. Waldo, and K. Levit. 1980. National health expenditures. *Health Care Financing Review.* 5:1-30.

Greenwald, H. P., M. Peterson, L. Garrison, et al. 1984. Interspeciality variation in office-based care. *Med. Care.* 22:14-29.

Grossman, R. M. 1983. A review of physician cost containment strategies for laboratory testing. *Medical Care.* 21(8):783.

Hoey, J., J. Eisenberg, W. Spitzer, and D. Thomas. 1982. Physicians sensitivity to the price of diagnostic tests: A U.S.-Canadian analysis. *Med. Care.* 20:302-307.

Knapp, D. E., D. Knapp, M. Speedie, D. Yaeger, and C. Baker. 1979. Relationship of inappropriate drug prescription to increased length of hospital stay. *American Journal of Hospital Pharmacy.* 36:1334-1337.

Long, M. J., K. Cummings, and K. Frisof. 1983. The role of perceived price in physicians demand for diagnostic tests. *Med. Care.* 21:243-250.

Maronde, R. F., P. Lee, M. McCarron, and S. Seibert. 1971. A study of prescribing patterns. *Med. Care.* 9:383-395.

McCarthy, E. G. and M. Finkel. Second opinion elective surgery programs: Outcome status over time. *Med. Care.* 16:984-994.

Mohr, J. W., ed. 1971. National survey of clinical labs. *Laboratory Management.* 9:17.

Noren, J., T. Frazier, I. Altman, and J. DeLozier. 1980. Ambulatory medical care: A comparison of internists and family—general practitioners. *New England Journal of Medicine.* 302:11-16.

Omachonu, V. K. and R. Nanda. 1988. IEs in health care management must emphasize client-centered projects which can contain cost while supporting quality. *Industrial Engineering*. Norcross, GA: Institute of Industrial Engineers. 20(10):66.

_____. 1988. A conceptual framework for hospital nursing unit productivity measurement. *Industrial Engineering*. Norcross, GA: Institute of Industrial Engineers. 20(5):56.

_____. 1988. A diagnosis-based approach to hospital nursing unit productivity measurement. *Proceedings, 9th Annual Conference*. American Society for Engineering Management. p. 251.

_____.1989. Measuring hospital nursing unit productivity under the new reimbursement scheme. *Productivity Management Frontiers II*. Sumanth, et al., eds. Switzerland: Inderscience Enterprises Ltd. p. 63.

Pineault, R. 1976. The effect of prepaid group practice on physicians utilization behavior. *Med. Care*. 14:121-136.

_____. 1977. The effect of medical training factors on physicians utilization behavior. *Med. Care*. 15:51-67.

Read, J. L., R. S. Stern, L. A. Thibodeau, D. E. Geer, Jr., D.E. and H. Klapholz. 1984. Variation in office-based care. *Med. Care*. 22:14-29.

Rhee, S. O., R. Luke, and Culverwell. 1980. Influence of client/colleague dependence on physician performance in patient care. *Med. Care*. 18:829-841.

Schroeder, S. A., A. Schliftman, and T. Piemm. 1974. Variation among physicians in use of laboratory tests: Relation to quality of care. *Med. Care*. 12:709-713.

Schroeder, S. A., L. Myers, and S. McPhee. 1984. The failure of physician education as a cost containment strategy: Report of a prospective controlled trial at a university hospital. *J.A.M.A.* 252:225-230.

Wennberg, J. E. and Gittelsohn. 1982. Variations in medical care among small areas. *Scientific American*. 246(4):120-134.

Wilensky, G. R. and L. Rossiter. 1983. The relative importance of physician-induced demand for medical care. *Milbank Mem. Fund Quarterly*. 61:252-277.

Young, W. and R. Saltman. 1982. Medical practice, case mix and cost containment: A new role for the attending physician. *J.A.M.A.* 247:801-805.

Zurker, B. ed. 1976. National survey of non-hospital clinical laboratories. *Laboratory Management*. 14(17).

Part Four

Achieving Quality and Productivity Through Technology and Engineering Management

This section examines the critical role of technology and engineering management in attaining quality, productivity, and competitiveness in the health-care industry.

Chapter Nine presents a detailed discussion on health-care technologies and the need for effective management. A working definition of technology management in health-care organizations is proposed, as well as an analysis of the role of clinical engineering.

In Chapter Ten, the role of health-care management engineers is examined in the context of total quality transformation. The chapter explores the specific skills that today's management engineers possess, which make their role essential in achieving the transformation of health-care organizations.

9 Technology Management in Health Care

As the preceding chapters have shown, the issues of quality, productivity, efficiency, effectiveness, and competitiveness have become more important today than ever before. Increasingly, hospitals are turning to technology as a vehicle for addressing these issues. As medical intervention takes on a multidimensional approach—one that draws upon the expertise of physicians, pharmacists, anesthesiologists, diagnostic technicians, materials services, clinical engineering, and nursing—the state of technology management becomes even more critical. The cost of technology remains a key issue for hospitals. Health care providers are compelled to balance the value of life against technology's strain on economic resources.

Since hospital management has become more complex, hospital administrators need an increasing number of technical specialists to provide expertise in various operational and decision-making areas. One such area is technical management. Today, a patient entering a hospital will most likely come in contact with one or more pieces of technical equipment: a patient monitor, respirator, electroencephalograph (EEG), heart pacemaker, electrocardiograph (ECG), high voltage radio therapy equipment, X-ray equipment, defibrillator, anesthesia machine, heart pump, dialysis machine, suction pump, hyperthermia apparatus, or heart-lung machine. Technological advances in the number, variety, and complexity of these devices create a need for effective management of hospital technology.

HEALTH-CARE TECHNOLOGIES

Health-care technologies can be classified primarily under the following four categories:

• diagnostic technology
• therapeutic technology
• information system technology
• multipurpose (combination) technology

Diagnostic technologies are primarily used for measuring and testing; *therapeutic technologies* are used directly for treating patients; *information system technologies* refer to technologies that support information (data) gathering, analysis, storage, and retrieval; and *multipurpose technologies* represent a combination of two or all of the other technologies. It should be noted that although diagnostic and therapeutic technologies are listed separately, they may contain built-in information system technologies. Table 9-1 shows examples of the technology categories.

It is important to understand how all four technology categories interact with the patient. Also of immense significance is the interaction between the technologies and the hospital environment, as depicted in Figure 9-1.

Today, more than any time before, the perception that the level of a hospital's technology is directly related to its quality of care, is gaining support among health-care clinicians and administrators. In a survey of 10,000 physicians in 100 hospitals, conducted by Professional Research Consultants Inc. (AHA News, 1988), 74 percent of the physicians surveyed said availability of new technology was a very important factor in their selection of hospitals for patients.

The increased role of biomedical engineering research is indicative of the steady growth of engineering and technology

Table 9-1. Types of health-care technologies.

Therapeutic Technology		Diagnostic Technology	
Examples: • Defibrillator • Pacemaker • Infusion device • Radiation therapy • Ventilators • Lasers • Incubators • Respirators	• Electrosurgical equipment • Hemodialysis machine • Heart-lung machine • Heart catheters • Resuscitators • Physical therapy equipment • Diathermy equipment	Examples • X-ray units • Cat-scanner • Fetal monitor • Cardiac monitor • Patient monitor • EEG • Recorder	• Automated blood analyzer • Hemotology equipment • Electromyrographs (EMG) • Gas chromatographs • Telemetry equipment • ECG
Information System Technology		**Multipurpose Technology**	
Examples : • Clinical information system with capability of automatically recording vital signs • Patient care planning infomation system, e.g., billing, appointments, and registration • Bedside terminals • Cost accounting system • Productivity monitoring system		Example: • A combination of a cardiac monitor, an infusion pump and a computer (attachment). Through programming, the diagnosis is obtained from the cardiac monitor, and the program automatically selects a course of treatment.	

in medicine. According to Khalil and Waly (1988), "Modern equipment, diagnostic techniques, surgery and therapy procedures are becoming increasingly dependent on recent developments in biomedical technology." The efforts of NASA, Bell Laboratory, and some private agencies have contributed immensely to the development of hospital technologies.

Technology has been actively adopted for its capacity to enhance health-care diagnostic, therapeutic, and information systems. Prior to the introduction of DRGs, there was little concern over the cost of hospital technologies, primarily because both consumers and providers could pass the costs along to willing third party payers. The introduction of DRGs has given rise to increased scrutiny, owing to the general concern over rising health-care costs.

Technology has the potential of increasing and decreasing health-care costs. A certain technology may raise the input to health-care costs while increasing manpower productivity or quality of service. An acceptable medium must be sought between these two competing consequences.

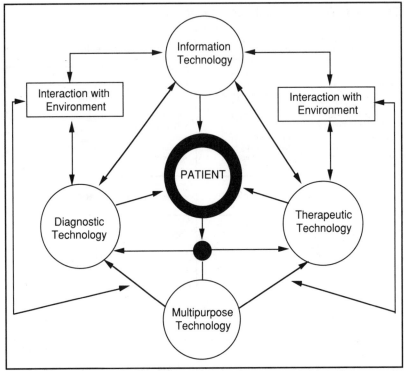

Figure 9-1. Hospital technology, the environment, and patient interaction.

DEFINITION OF TECHNOLOGY MANAGEMENT IN HEALTH-CARE ORGANIZATIONS

The technology of a health-care organization is a difficult subject to address because it means different things to different people. There exists a widely divergent spectrum of opinions from clinicians, researchers, administrators, and other health-care technical groups as to what constitutes hospital technology. To most people in the health-care industry, technology plays a vital role in increasing an organization's efficiency, bringing about or facilitating the process of recovery, pinpointing the cause of illness more accurately, finding a cure, etc.

Technology management as discussed in this book is based on technology in terms of equipment, instrumentation, and devices employed in care delivery. These features are immediately controllable at the hospital level. Issues such as vaccine development, drugs, artificial body parts, cancer research, and AIDS research are not addressed in this book. Based on this premise, the following definition is given:

> *Technology management in health-care organizations involves the coordination, maintenance and integration of diverse technological systems that support the health-care delivery process, structure, and outcome, through the activities of prepurchase planning, purchasing, maintenance, and evaluation, with a view to ensuring quality, competitiveness, and cost containment. Prepurchase planning includes information gathering to determine needs, selection process, bids solicitation, obtaining references from users, system integration design, space allocation, and cost of ownership. Purchasing deals with the actual acquisition and training needs. Maintenance is concerned with the implementation of preventive maintenance and corrective maintenance programs, contracted maintenance service, and shared maintenance service. Evaluation is aimed at examining the present status of each technology with respect to the whole, in order to address the issues of suitability, impact on quality, upgradeability, replacement, lease or buy options, etc.*

Figure 9-2 shows the health-care technology management cycle. The cycle depicts a continuous process with built-in improvement activities.

The factors that affect technology management in health-care organizations are complex and sometimes difficult to define. Figure 9-3 represents an attempt to integrate all of these macro factors into what is called a conceptual framework for managing technology. As a general rule, all activities resulting from a well-balanced technology management policy should lead directly to the organization's short-term and long-term goals.

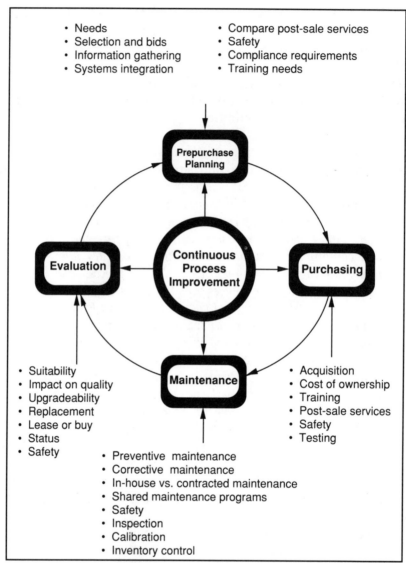

Figure 9-2. The health-care technology management cycle.

THE ROLE OF CLINICAL/BIOMEDICAL ENGINEERING

Fundamental to the creation of clinical engineering is the notion that technology without the appropriate hands-on technologists to manage it is doomed to fail. This rationale explains the emergence of an entirely new profession in the late 1960s called

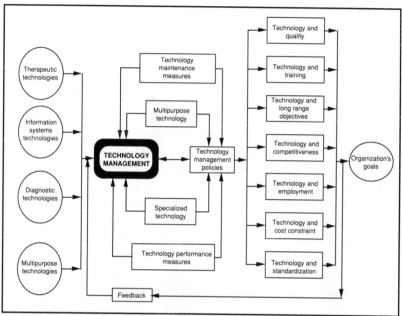

Figure 9-3. A conceptual framework for the management of technology in health-care organizations.

clinical engineering (also called biomedical engineering). Clinical engineering seeks to serve as the liaison between health care and the increasingly complex technologies supporting it. The principal responsibility of the clinical engineering department is to coordinate the application of technology as it is used for diagnosis, therapy, information gathering and analysis, or any combination thereof. Clinical engineering activities typically include consultation in instrument selection and purchase, planned maintenance programs, safety testing, instrument calibration and repair, and managing equipment insurance and educational services.

Even now, the role of clinical engineering is not fully understood by hospital administrators. In fact, many administrators do not know what a clinical engineer is. The general perception is that clinical engineering only deals with the repair of equipment. While the perception may have been valid two or three decades ago, today's need to manage the interaction among diverse technologies, health-care personnel, and patients has caused clinical engineering to play a broader role. The specific responsibilities of clinical engineering are listed below:

Prepurchase evaluation. Clinical engineering works in conjunction with the nursing and medical staffs to evaluate the safety and operating effectiveness of all medical equipment used for patient care. This necessitates the need to develop appropriate specifications for competitive bidding when new equipment needs to be purchased. A critical evaluation must be made of the various equipment on the market and their uses. Considerations as to equipment and reliability and performance history should also be investigated by the clinical engineering department. Selection of the most suitable equipment can save time and money as a result of shorter time required to train users, reduced frequency of breakdowns and accompanying inconveniences, shorter intervals of inactivity while equipment is being fixed, etc. If purchasing decisions are made by nontechnical individuals, the purchased equipment may be incompatible with the environment in which its use is intended. It is not uncommon to find a costly and sophisticated device being abused or misused, thus causing further service problems for the biomedical technician or clinical engineer.

In equipment selection, special consideration should also be given to cost of ownership (installed cost), space requirement, location, and the total system requirement (compatibility with existing systems). A complete analysis of all life cycle costs will be useful to hospital administrators in determining the best equipment for their purpose.

Incoming inspections. Clinical engineering is responsible for conducting incoming inspections on all new, trial, loaner, leased, rental, demonstration, or privately owned instrumentation or equipment to be used for patient care.

Service and repairs. Response time to requests for services is a vital component of a clinical engineering department. Such requests typically originate from departments where the equipment is located, and depending on the nature of the request, clinical engineering may elect to conduct an initial evaluation and then assign some priority (based on availability of resources) to the task.

Preventive maintenance. This involves establishing protocols and schedules for periodical inspections to ensure conformance to manufacturers' specifications and compliance with existing standards and codes.

In-service training. A regular training program is often maintained for the clinical staff and other users of various state-of-the-art medical technologies.

Inventory control. Records for all equipment should be maintained showing each piece's complete history, repairs, names of all technicians who have worked on the equipment, costs of materials and labor, and other reports of use.

Equipment insurance program. Clinical engineering manages equipment insurance provided by specialty underwriters.

Device acquisition. The device procurement process begins with the articulation of a need and ends when a justifiable need is completely and satisfactorily met. Clinical engineering serves as the liaison between the department initiating the request, the purchasing department, and the device manufacturer. Whitworth (1980) notes that "All hospital staff want equipment, to replace current outdated equipment, to perform some function for which equipment has not previously been available, to provide essential benefits and nice-to-have benefits. And always, the equipment wanted is more than can be afforded and in competition with those items wanted by others. The clinical engineer working with the user and purchasing department has a vital role to play in educating the user about the most efficient and economical ways to meet his or her needs." Figure 9-4 depicts the procurement process.

In-House Repair and Maintenance Service

The primary objective of setting up an in-house repair and maintenance support system is to provide the equipment user with a service that is equal to or better than the service provided by the equipment manufacturer or other third parties. Three principal criteria are used to make the assessment: quality of

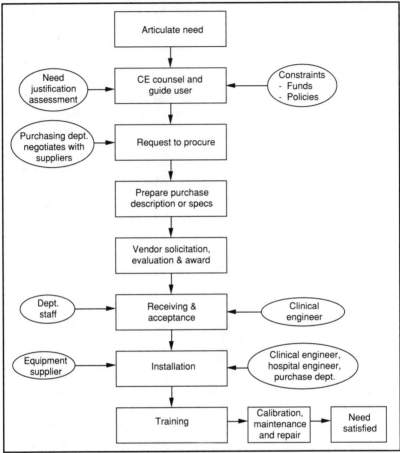

Figure 9-4. The procurement process.

technical support, response time for service requests, and cost of providing the service. An in-house repair and maintenance program must satisfy all three of these criteria.

Quality Considerations

As stated in Chapter Four, there are two components of service quality: technical quality and perceived quality. Since clinical engineering offers a service, its quality should be evaluated on the basis of both the soft and hard factors of quality. The perceived quality components (soft factors) include speed of response to a problem and attitude toward the problem.

While these two factors have nothing to do with the ability of clinical engineering to solve a problem effectively, they are a basis for the service recipient's perceived quality. The faster a person can respond to a problem, the better the perceived quality becomes. Most health-care providers depend very heavily on technology, and their perceived level of quality is influenced by the time it takes to receive requested equipment and the time it takes to solve the problem.

Attitude, on the other hand, involves professionalism, appearance, manners, courtesy, and sensitivity to the user's problems. Boxerman (1980) reports the results of a survey of hospital administrators whose hospitals have an in-house clinical engineering department. According to the survey, 61 percent of the administrators said that the most important quality of a clinical engineer is the ability to get along with people.

All of these *soft* factors combine to create the notion of quality in the mind of the user. It should be pointed out, however, that quality on the basis of the soft factors is a necessary but not sufficient condition for overall service excellence. The technical quality component must be sufficiently present for true overall quality service to exist.

The hard factor in perceived quality is the technical competency of the clinical engineering staff. Technical competency is reflected in the service technician's knowledge of the user's equipment and how it functions. Multiple unsuccessful attempts to repair the same or what appears to be the same problem quickly diminishes the perceived quality of the service.

TECHNOLOGY MAINTENANCE PROGRAMS

Health-care technologies, like other technologies, wear out with use and thus need repairs and replacement. Maintenance is the function that keeps health-care delivery systems operable. Aimed at keeping or restoring any piece of medical technology operating satisfactorily, it usually involves such tasks as replacing worn-out parts, servicing equipment, inspections, making emergency repairs, and so forth. Without proper maintenance, costs such as excessive idle time and unsafe working conditions could be experienced.

The maintenance function may be centralized, decentralized, or a combination of both. With centralization, the biomedical technicians/clinical engineers are in one location and are assigned responsibilities as need arises. Decentralization allows workers to be located in different areas of the hospital, and responsibilities are confined to those areas. The extent to which decentralization occurs depends on the following:

- the specific demand for maintenance services
- the travel (or response) time between the piece of equipment and the central shop
- the seriousness (cost) of downtime
- the degree of specialization required

While centralization results in a more efficient use of personnel, decentralization results in faster service. Maintenance costs tend to be lower when a piece of equipment is new and increase as they grow older. The major operational choice for clinical/biomedical engineering is whether to repair equipment before it malfunctions (preventive maintenance) or wait until it malfunctions before repairing it (breakdown or corrective maintenance). Although preventive measures do not stop breakdowns, they do reduce them. Preventive maintenance requires planning and scheduling of activities, while breakdown maintenance is said to be management by exception. The best type of maintenance policy to adopt is the one that provides the lowest total cost. Typical breakdown costs include:

- repairs
- equipment/instrumentation downtime
- idle labor (nurses, physicians, technicians)
- loss of output
- schedule delays
- customer dissatisfaction (patients, nurses, physicians)

Although in the mid-1970s, the Joint Commission on Accreditation of Hospitals (JCAHO) mandated the use of preventive maintenance programs on medical equipment, its benefits have not been fully understood by health-care practitioners.

The benefits that can be derived from a well designed and well managed preventive maintenance program include:

- reduced cost of repairs
- decreased downtime due to failures
- extended equipment life
- increased customer satisfaction
- reduced severity and frequency of equipment failures
- increased equipment performance, safety, and working condition
- reduced incidents of output loss
- decreased idle labor

Key Elements of a Preventive Maintenance Program

Preventive maintenance means routine servicing and inspections to detect potential failure conditions and to make corrections that will prevent major problems. It is most effective when failures can be predicted with some accuracy. Critical to a preventive maintenance program is anticipating key difficulties and then performing the expected repairs before they are actually needed. Preventive maintenance is generally desirable when it can increase the operating time of an asset by reducing severity or frequency of breakdowns. In hospitals, preventive maintenance typically includes cleaning, inspection, lubricating, calibration, testing, complete overhauls, or the replacement of critical parts before failure.

As a general rule, if an equipment failure may result in harm to a patient or employee, a wrong diagnosis, stopping the care delivery process, or wasting the hospital's resources (assets), then it should be considered for preventive maintenance.

As the health-care delivery process relies more and more on technology, maintenance increases in significance. Effective preventive maintenance requires adequately trained personnel, a good equipment record system, properly defined procedures for preventive maintenance inspections, and planned maintenance schedules.

Equipment record system. Pertinent information on each piece of equipment, such as description, model and serial number, manufacturer, acquisition costs, location, vendor, contract number, date of acquisition, equipment purpose, hospital asset number, etc. should be recorded. This record should be updated as each piece of equipment is updated, serviced, rebuilt, or replaced. Good maintenance records provide substantial assistance in estimating the probabilistic distributions of breakdown and repair times. The essential items of an effective equipment maintenance records system are presented in Figures 9-5 and 9-6.

Equipment Maintenance Records (EMR) Systems

Equipment name:	Model:	Serial number:	Manufacturer:	Vendor:
Purchase date:	Department of user:	Location of equipment:	Contract number:	Acquisition Cost:
Purchase order number:	Year introduced:	Space requirement (sq .feet):	Warranty period:	Preventive maintenance schedule:
What equipment is used for :		Preventive maintenance procedure (summary) :		
YTD labor cost:	YTD material cost:	Approx. training time required:	Process rate:	

Figure 9-5. Equipment maintenance records systems by device.

Order #	Asset #	Date of Service Requisition	Date of Response	Equipment Name / Location	Nature of Work	Service Completion Date	Technician's Name	Labor Hours (min/hrs)	Outcome
					e. g. : • Performance inspection • Unit rebooked • Unit cleaned • Diagnostics performed • Vendor coordinated repair work				

Figure 9-6. Equipment maintenance records system by service provided.

Preventive maintenance inspection procedures. Although most equipment manufacturers provide certain procedures for conducting the required preventive maintenance, such procedures tend to be too technical, complex, and sometimes impractical. An efficient clinical engineering department should develop its own procedures for preventive maintenance.

Planned maintenance schedule. In theory, the optimum preventive maintenance schedule is one that minimizes that device's total maintenance costs and downtime. Unlike most industries, hospitals are a seven-day week business, unaffected by holidays, weekends, etc. It is usually difficult to find a convenient time to perform a preventive maintenance activity. There are no general rules on whether to schedule preventive maintenance weekly, monthly, quarterly, etc. The following factors are helpful, however, when developing a preventive maintenance schedule:

• impact of equipment function and failure
• equipment volume, type, complexity, and location
• equipment availability
• requirements of regulatory agencies
• frequency of use
• age of equipment

Adequate training. Today's health-care technologies are more sophisticated and complex than ever before. It used to be that a technician with moderate training, could perform repairs by referring to a service manual. The manuals, like the technology, have become more complicated and confusing, requiring a more sophisticated level of training for the maintenance staff. Training should be an on-going process if the preventive maintenance program is not to be compromised.

Training Requirements

It is important to note that nurses are the primary users of hospital equipment and many of them feel inadequately trained in the use of some equipment. Barger, et al. (1980) reported the results of a survey conducted to determine the level of nursing competence on 30 common equipment items. Twenty-five percent of the nurses surveyed felt that their knowledge of defibrillators and electrocardiogram monitors was either poor or incomplete, and 33 percent felt their knowledge of respirators was inadequate. It is estimated that approximately 80 percent of service calls received by the clinical engineering department can be attributed to the user's incomplete understanding of how to use a piece of equipment. Although training is generally provided by the hospital and by the equipment manufacturers, it is often inadequate. Some problems commonly associated with many training programs available today are presented below.

Labor turnover rate. The high labor turnover rate in nursing in particular, and other related health-care disciplines, tends to diminish the effectiveness of training programs. Medical technologies change very rapidly and there are usually different versions of a particular technology from competing manufacturers. Consequently, changing jobs from one hospital to another often creates the need to be retrained in the use of a different version of an already familiar technology.

Training methods. Several methods are being used for on- and off-site training. They include face-to-face teaching, print or non-print materials or a combination of these. Figure 9-7 shows the results of a survey of training methods used by ambulatory care centers.

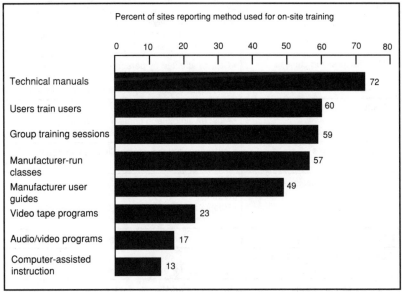

Figure 9-7. Ambulatory care centers' methods of on-site training for medical equipment. *(Source: U.S. Healthcare, November, 1989.)*

The suitability of a particular training method depends on several factors such as the equipment type, complexity of the process, technical background of users, etc. No one training method is best for all situations. The problems commonly associated with the various training methods are summarized in Table 9-2.

COMPUTER INFORMATION SYSTEMS TECHNOLOGY

The switch to a DRG system and the prospective payment system has led to heavy dependency on data. The need to comply with the quality assurance requirements of JCAHO as well as to meet or surpass the customers' expectations has given birth to detailed documentation requirements. The volume and quality of data now associated with providing health care has made manual methods of data collection, manipulation, storage, and retrieval nearly untenable. Today's computer information technology argues forcefully for an integrated computer

Table 9-2. Problems associated with training methods.

Training Method	Possible Problems
1.Technical manuals	• Sometimes too technical, confusing, intimidating, and not adequately illustrated. • People generally dislike manuals and would avoid using them if possible.
2.Manufacturer-run classes	• Can be affected by personnel changes, unless offered regularly. • May require travel to the manufacturer's facility.
3.Manufacturer user guides	• Sometimes too technical. • Must be simple and contain adequate diagrammatic illustrations to be effective.
4.Users train users	• Improperly trained users will teach improper methods to others.
5.Group training sessions	• Effectiveness diminishes with excessively large groups. • People are sometimes too embarrassed to ask questions in group settings.
6.Video tape programs	May require additional cost for viewing equipment.
7.Computer assisted instructions	Not suitable for every piece of medical equipment.
8.Audio/video programs	May require additional cost for viewing equipment.

system to provide information in a timely manner, thereby improving the effectiveness and efficiency of clinical practice. Computer applications most frequently used in care facilities include those for registration, patient billing, medical records, physician billing, accounts receivable, and patient scheduling.

Computer information systems can positively affect the health-care delivery process in several ways. For example, implementation of a computer information system may improve

• the timeliness of patient care due to reduced turn around time for test results.
• the speed, quality, and presentation of test reports to physicians.
• the data base required to support the quality assurance programs and instruments.
• the tracking of resource quantities consumed (by DRGs, nursing unit, day, shift, etc.).
• the management controls for cost containment, such as total productivity and DRG-based productivity programs.

Pre-computerization Analysis

The decision to computerize a hospital's information system should begin with a clear and concise definition of the problem. Once defined, the problem should be analyzed, alternatives should be sought out, evaluated, and the best one recommended. Table 9-3 summarizes the process of pre-computerization analysis.

Table 9-3. Factors to consider during pre-computerization analysis.

1. Problem definition	Clear and concise statement of the problem.
2. Problem analysis	Who will be affected by the problem? How does the problem impact quality of patient care? What causes the problem? What is the extent of the problem?
3. Search for possible alternatives	How can the objectives be accomplished? What other options are available other than computerization?
4. Evaluate alternatives	a) Fiscal considerations: 　Cost of the project (installed) 　• Hardware 　• Software 　• Personnel 　• Training 　• Operating and maintenance 　• Expected savings b) Technical considerations: 　• What level of technical know-how is needed to run the system? 　• Can the system be integrated with the other technical systems in the organization? 　• What are the prospects for upgradeability? c) Organizational considerations: 　• How will the system affect the structure of the organization, information flow, organizational culture, and ethics? 　• Is resistance to change a major factor and how will it be dealt with? 　• Will the system affect the balance of power in the organization? d) Staff considerations: 　• How will the system affect staff size? 　• If staff reduction is inevitable, what provisions can be made for other placements? 　• What training needs will be created? 　• What new staff specialities will be needed and how will they be obtained? e) Legal considerations: 　• What are the legal ramifications in the adoption or acquisition of a given plan? 　• What is the cost of compliance or legal support? 　• What are the prospects of lawsuits? f) Security considerations: 　• What security risks can be associated with the system? 　• What will be the cost of risk minimization? g) Patient considerations: 　• How will the system affect quality of care (quality of conformance and perceived quality)? 　• How will the system affect the cost of patient care? h) Competition considerations: 　• What competitive advantages will be derived by acquiring this system?
5. Recommendation	What is the recommendation that will best compliment the short- and long-term goals of the organization, while satisfying the present constraints of the organization?

Developing a Computer Information System for Hospitals

Developing of a hospital computer information system should begin with a thorough analysis to identify the needs, drawing input from the potential users of the information to be generated. Once agreement has been reached on the needs of these users, the process of classifying and collecting data begins. Various instruments are utilized for data collection, including forms, files, surveys, etc. This is followed by data recording, sorting and stratification, and finally communicating the output to the users. Figure 9-8 provides a flowchart of the process.

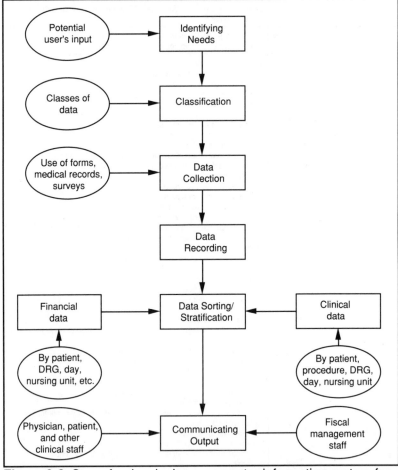

Figure 9-8. Steps for developing a computer information system for hospitals.

Computer Information Systems and Organizational Changes

Undoubtedly, introducing computers into a health-care environment can create significant impacts, including changes in work methods, establishment of new procedures, reorganization of work units, and hiring of new employees. Data processing activities, including the appearance of new computer terminals, will be very noticeable. New terms such as "data base," "software," "hardware," "fields," "on-line," and "management information systems" will become prevalent throughout the work place. Leadership will also be affected—either at the unit level, department level, or hospital-wide. According to Boettinger (1970), "One can compensate for bad technology to some extent with great leadership and for poor leadership with superb technology. But peak performance can never be achieved without peaks in both domains—the human and the technical." Listed below are some of the organizational changes which may occur as a result of installing a computer information system.

Role changes. In some cases, computerization may necessitate changes in roles. Nursing, for example, may be responsible for certain activities which, after the installation of a computerized information system, are performed more efficiently by other departments. Another key area where changes can be anticipated is management information systems (MIS). The customers of MIS are health-care managers and administrators. These customers perceive MIS to be the source of information and data for decision making. Health care managers depend on MIS for timely and accurate information. In the context of total quality management, health-care administrators are looking at data over time, to help them identify special causes of variations. Rather than receive pages filled with numbers from MIS, health-care managers now expect to receive "run charts," control charts, and other reports that will directly support the goals of TQM. TQM requires MIS specialists not only to supply raw data, but to make sense out of them in terms of quality management.

Staff additions. The new system may create the need for new positions. In the laboratory, for example, a new person may be needed to enter test results into the system.

Resisting new responsibilities. Computerization may also necessitate shifts in responsibilities among departments and individuals. A department may resist taking on these newly assigned responsibilities which had been previously borne by another department.

Computer skills. Employees already possessing computer skills may be asked to interact with the new computer system more than those who do not already possess such skills.

Communication. With the new system, most communication will be accomplished via the computer, reducing communication among individuals, particularly telephone communications.

Individual responsibilities. Individual responsibilities may be reduced as a result of computer information support. This may decrease the skill level required by the affected positions.

Decision-making. The new computer information system may improve the decision-making capability of health-care administrators, by providing accurate and timely information.

Test results reporting. Test results should be created, analyzed, and reported faster due to the loss of administrative time involved. This includes physician's orders, radiology and laboratory results, and staff communications.

Time savings. More nursing time can be spent on direct patient care as the system is learned. Less time will be needed for clerical functions as the system's capabilities are learned.

Patient waiting time. A computer information system can, to a large extent, reduce patient waiting time during admission, test ordering, ancillary services ordering, meal selection, and discharge processing.

MANAGING RESISTANCE TO CHANGE

Dowling (1980) surveyed a randomly selected sample of 40 public and private hospitals to study the evidence of resistance to computers. He estimated that staff resistance to, and interference with, computerized information systems has occurred in nearly half of the hospitals that have attempted to implement such systems. Resistance consists of any number of acts, deliberate or subconscious, that interfere with the effective implementation and/or use of a computerized application. Resistance to change can take the form of physical sabotage of computer equipment, absenteeism, lateness, work slowdowns, data tampering, and more.

The primary reasons for resistance to computers are listed below:

- Computers are often associated with layoffs and unemployment.

- Computers can be ego-threatening and intimidating. A clinically influential member of the nursing, medical, or administrative staff who is computer illiterate may fear a loss of respect and status in the organization if computers are used.

- Workers may fear a loss of power due to transfer of functions that they used to perform.

- Some professionals fear that computers are too impersonal, inflexible, and structured.

- Fear of having to learn something new may create extra pressure.

Dealing with Resistance to Change

The following guidelines are recommended for dealing with resistance to change:

- Involve staff from the beginning when considering introducing a computer system.

- Reassure the staff that their interests and needs will be reflected in the design of the system.

- Train and educate staff prior to system start-up.

- Vigorously sell the computerization concept to all involved. Present proof from studies indicating the potential benefits from the new system.

- Discuss potential problems as well as the positive implications of the new system with the staff, and jointly develop ways of overcoming problems.

- Arrange for continuous training sessions, learning aids, and help sources to facilitate use of the system.

- Encourage feedback and address each concern expressed by the users of the system.

- Ergonomically design each workstation to insure user safety and comfort.

Systems Integration and New Technologies

For hospitals and health service providers, integrated systems have become an operational necessity. In addition to reducing paperwork and costs, they provide the government and private payers, such as insurance companies, vital statistics on patients and costs. Integrated systems also help health organizations comply with a myriad of federal, state, and local regulations. Some of today's more sophisticated systems handle information on patient care and integrate communications among doctors, nurses, and ancillary hospital departments.

Fifty health-care providers surveyed reported spending an average of $25 million on information systems yearly, growing at a rate of 7.6 percent annually (Avery 1990). These systems are often referred to by names such as patient care management systems (which integrate the functions of billing, accounting, scheduling and patient monitoring) and nursing management systems (which handle initial assessments of patients and plans for their care, and records and organizes progress notes and information generated from bedside point-of-care terminals).

Other new technologies such as smart cards are also emerging into the health-care scene. Smart cards are plastic cards (developed primarily for patient registration) with a magnetic or optical strip containing general information. Another technology that has been used, with limited success in health care, is artificial intelligence.

TECHNOLOGY MANAGEMENT AND DECISION MAKING LATITUDE

Owing to the multi-disciplinary nature of health care, decision making authority is somewhat diffused among the following key players:

- CEO/administrator
- Chief financial officer
- Hospital governing board
- Chief medical director
- Director of nursing
- Chief purchasing officer
- Department manager/head
- Materials services
- Clinical/biomedical engineering

Traditionally, most of the decision making authority was in the hands of physicians. Today, many hospitals are beginning to utilize administrative councils, program committees, and strategic management teams to oversee and manage modern technological systems. The increasing number of clinicians and administrators with technical and business degrees is expected to cause the decision making latitude to become further diffused. In a survey in which 250 hospital CEOs were asked which factors were the most important in the decision to purchase a new technology, 52% said physicians' preference, 25.6% said cost, 9.2% said competition, and 13.2% were uncertain (*Hospitals* 1989).

When deciding to purchase new medical technology, the following topics should be discussed:

- purchasing of technological systems
- replacing and/or adopting new technology
- scrapping old or existing technological programs
- making lease or buy decisions
- research and development priorities
- sharing technology between facilities
- specialized or multipurpose technologies
- upgrading existing technologies

Today, physicians, nurses, and other technical staff are responsible for developing proposals for new technologies which are evaluated by various administrative councils. Under the present system of fixed (DRG) reimbursement rates, such proposals must now contain cost justifications and clearly detailed statements of benefits and expenses. Clinicians are now required to define what the new technology will do and purchasing is expected to solicit objective bids. Figure 9-9 depicted an example of the breakdown of the decision making influences involved in purchasing a medical records systems.

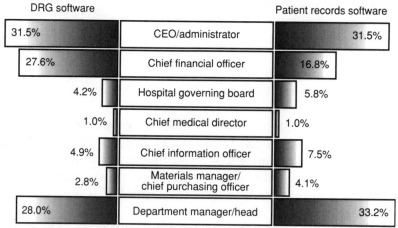

Figure 9-9. Purchasing decision for medical records systems.
(Reprinted from Buying Influences in Hospitals, by permission, Copyright 1988, American Hospital Publishing, Inc.)

Listed below are ten key questions for evaluating existing hospital technologies and potential upgrades or additions to the system.

1. Are training and employment issues adequately addressed with respect to a total systems technology?

2. From a systems viewpoint, are the technologies compatible with the long range objectives of the organization ?

3. Is quality of care the central focus of the systems' technologies?

4. Are the technologies compatible with the organization's competitiveness goals?

5. Are cost considerations (purchasing, operating, maintenance, installation and pay back) fully considered in the selection of a given technology?

6. Is there a properly established channel for obtaining information regarding new and state-of-the-art technologies and also for matching the user's clinical and environmental needs with the existing technologies?

7. Are there policies in place for training, upkeep, modernization, upgradeability, replacement, etc., of technologies?

8. Is there a formal process for monitoring the performance of the "technology management department," as well as each piece of technology? (Performance monitoring should include percent utilization, efficiency, effectiveness, impact on quality, accuracy of readings, failure or breakdown rates, reliability, maintenance cost as a percent of acquisition cost, percentage of same-day response, etc.)

9. Does the hospital have a committee, or department charged with the responsibility of technology management?

10. Is formal attention given to the issues of safety (accident

prevention), risk management, confidentiality of results and information, backup for critical technologies in case of failure, and cooperation between the technology manufacturer (or provider) and the user?

EXERCISES

9-1. A local hospital classifies its technology as diagnostic, therapeutic, information systems, and multipurpose, respectively. The table is used to gather figures for corrective maintenance, preventive maintenance, acquisition costs, and installation costs for each category of the technology.

	Corrective Maintenance		Preventive Maintenance		Acquisition		Installation	
	Costs	%	Costs	%	Costs	%	Costs	%
Diagnostic Technology								
Therapeutic Technology								
Information Systems Technology								
Multipurpose Technology								
Total Annual Cost								

Perform an analysis of your hospital's costs and record them in the table provided, using only technology that you have owned for at least one year. What can you deduce from this analysis? What effects would the age of the respective technologies have on your analysis and conclusions?

9-2. Suppose that your hospital currently employs three training techniques to teach your staff how to use its available technologies. The techniques are technical manuals, users training users, and video tape. Design an experiment to study the effectiveness of each training program in terms of the following:

- frequency of calls for help by trained staff
- reasons for calls by trained staff
- time elapsed since training occurred
- training method preference

Conduct this study at your facility. What conclusions can be made from your results?

9-3. The following information has been gathered from a local hospital.

Equipment Type	Equipment Age	Number of calls per month
1. Hemodialysis medicine	12 months	2
2. Defibrillator	22 months	5
3. Cat-scanner	43 months	4
4. Cardiac monitor	18 months	3
5. Automated blood analyzer	27 months	7
. . .	. . .	. . .
. . .	. . .	. . .
. . .	. . .	. . .

Perform a similar analysis at your facility. What conclusions can you draw from the data you have collected? What implications are there for a technology management policy?

BIBLIOGRAPHY

Adamson, H. W. 1982. Evolution of a hospital-based clinical engineering contract service. *Journal of Clinical Engineering.* 7(4):313-315.

AHA News. 1988. Staff quality is critical factor in admitting. July 18. p.8.

Avery, C. 1990. Treating the whole. *Complete System News.* Jan. 22. p. 31.

Barger, M., C. Bandy, P. Marcus, and S. Padow. 1980. The acquisition and maintenance of medical equipment. *Management and Clinical Engineering.* C. A. Caceres, ed. Dedham, NH: Artech House, Inc.

Boettinger, H. M. 1970. Technology in the manager's future. *Harvard Business Review.* Nov.-Dec. 48:4.

Bouley, A. J. and A. O'Brien. 1986. Clinical engineering and quality assurance. *Biomedical Technology Today.* 1(2):39-41.

Boxerman, S. B. 1980. The employers' perceptions of needs. *Management and Clinical Engineering.* C. A. Caceres, ed. Dedham, MA: Artech House, Inc.

Caceres, C. A., D. C. Hanlin, and J. L. Williams. 1980. The roots of clinical engineering. *Management and Clinical Engineering.* C. A. Caceres, ed. Dedham, MA: Artech House, Inc.

Dodson, B., A. Janke, G. Goodman, and G. Gordon. 1980. BMETs-The need for well trained support staff. *Management and Clinical Engineering.* C. A. Caceres, ed. Dedham, MA: Artech House, Inc.

Dowling, A. F. 1980. Hospital staff interfere with computer system implementation. *Health Care Management Review.* Fall, vol. 23.

Egdahl, R. H. and P. Gertman. 1978. *Technology and Quality of Health Care.* Germantown, MD: Aspen Publishing.

Fennigkoh, L. 1987. *Management of the Clinical Engineering Department.* Quest Publishing Company, Inc.

Fowler, G. 1985. Hospital sells its engineering services. *Hospitals.* 59(18):37.

Furst, E. Productivity and cost-effectiveness of clinical engineering. *Journal of Clinical Engineering.* 11:105-113.

Hager, D. E. 1981. Computers affect hospital organization, staff, patients. *Managing Computers in Health Care.* J. B. Worthley, ed. Ann Arbor, MI: AUPHA Press.

Hallock, R. I. 1979. With computers administrative attitude is the key to success. *Administrative Management.* March, vol. 80.

Hargest, T. S. 1980. Clinical engineering and nursing: An amiable marriage. *Management and Clinical Engineering,* C. A. Caceres, ed. Dedham, MA: Artech House, Inc.

Khalil, T. M. and Waly, S. M. 1988. Planning for health care technology transfer. *Technology Management I.* T. M. Khalil, et al., eds. Switzerland: Inderscience Enterprises, Ltd.

Ladsen, M. 1981. Turning reluctant users on to change. *Computer Decisions.* Jan. pp. 93-100.

Omachonu, V. K. 1990. Technology management in hospitals. *Management of Technology II.* T. M. Khalil and B. Bayraktar, eds. Norcross, GA: Institute of Industrial Engineers.

Omachonu, V. K. and R. Nanda. 1988. Developing a new data base for productivity information management. *Proceedings of the 10th Annual Computers and Industrial Engineering Conference.* 15:277.

_____. 1988. Developing an information base for measuring nursing unit productivity. *1988 IIE Integrated Systems Conference Proceedings.* Norcross, GA: Institute of Industrial Engineers.

_____. 1988. Hospital information technology management under the prospective pricing system. *Technology Management I.* T. M. Khalil, et al, eds. Switzerland: Inderscience Enterprises, Ltd.

_____. 1989. Measuring hospital nursing unit productivity under the new reimbursement system. *Productivity Management Frontiers II.* Switzerland: Inderscience Enterprises, Ltd.

Schmitz, H. 1977. A protocol for evaluating hospital information systems. *Hospital and Health Services Administration.* Winter 22:45-56.

Shafer, M. J., J. Carr, and M. Gordon. 1979. Clinical engineering—An enigma in health care facilities. *Hospital and Health Services Administration.* Summer. pp. 77-97.

Stewart, M. M. 1981. A better life through medical technology. *Medical Technology, Health Care and the Consumer.* Speigel, et al., eds. New York: Human Sciences Press.

Whitworth, D. P. 1980. Device acquisition. *Management and Clinical Engineering.* C. A. Caceres, ed. Dedham, MA: Artech House, Inc.

Worthley, J. A. 1981. *Managing Computers in Health Care.* Ann Arbor, MI: AUPHA Press.

10 The Role of Management Engineers in TQM

Health care is primarily a growth industry and some evidence of this can be found in the increasing emphasis on technological development, clinical capability, and greater reliance on the pure sciences. Accomplishments in all of these areas have been accompanied by rising costs. As the gap widens between consumer expectations and the services hospitals can deliver, health-care administrators are searching for ways to close this gap through more efficient resource management and quality improvement. The need is greater today for efficient management of human and non-human resources at all levels of a constrained hospital environment.

Industrial engineers (IEs), or management engineers as they have been commonly called, have been responding to this challenge by using basic techniques such as time study, activity sampling, and operations research tools for problem solving. Although these problem-solving tools can be effective in the process of continuous improvement, management engineers have generally used them to achieve the goals of cost containment rather than quality improvement. The role of today's management engineers needs to be redefined. Its definition must be based on a new paradigm of health-care practice—one that emphasizes quality improvement rather than arbitrary cost reductions. Without the adoption of a new operating philosophy, it will be difficult to realize the full benefits of the involvement of management engineers in the quality transformation (see Figure 10-1).

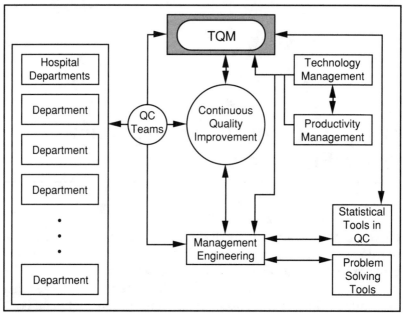

Figure 10-1. Management engineering interface with TQM.

Today's Perspective

There are between 4,000 and 5,000 IEs in the health care field today, many of whom are engaged in performing traditional IE-type functions. In a bid to remain economically viable, many hospitals have resorted to cost cutting measures such as personnel layoffs and departmental closings.

Among the most adversely affected personnel are management engineers. Sometimes the cost cutting measures are less drastic and the management engineering staffs are reassigned to other non IE-related functions. Presented below are several factors that contribute to this situation:

- identity problem
- internal hospital politics
- expendability of functions
- competition with external consultants
- conflicting and unclear roles
- new nursing initiatives
- new needs

Identity problem. Industrial engineers in hospitals have been experiencing an identity crisis since the 1950s when hospitals began to use IEs. Over the years, hospitals have resisted the idea of being seen as businesses or job shops. This resistance is partly responsible for the reluctance of hospitals to be associated with a field whose title is industrial engineering. As a result, IEs in hospitals are often referred to as management engineers, management services staff, technology managers, but never industrial engineers.

Perhaps even more critical is the fact that management engineers have not done enough to make themselves champions of the customers' concerns. Many members of the clinical staff often see management engineers as "the guys" who find reasons and ways to cut staff. This perception hardly makes management engineers advocates of customer satisfaction, or for that matter, champions of quality.

Hospital policies. Management engineering departments in hospitals are commonly perceived as the "omniscient" department that tells all other departments how inefficient they are. This misconception has been further reinforced by the countless management engineering studies documenting inefficiencies and ultimately resulting in manpower reduction and/or major reorganizations in administrative departments. Adverse political atmospheres have worsened since the implementation of the prospective payment reimbursement system.

Expendability of function. Unlike nurses, doctors, and admission clerks whose functions seem to be continuously needed, management engineers often find themselves entangled in the contemptuous role of fighting the question of expendability of their functions. The main thrust of management engineering activities has been in the area of staff support services, such as scheduling, time and motion studies, staffing, and facility design and location.

The general misconception is that there exists a finite number of management engineering studies to be undertaken in a hospital; once those studies are complete, the management engineering functions then become expendable. This accounts for one of the reasons why management engineers are the first people to go at a time of economic crisis. This idea defies the philosophy of continuous quality improvement. Quality improvement is a never-ending process.

Competition with external consultants. In general, management engineers in hospitals are often perceived as internal consultants whose services are needed only when problems arise. As a result of this perception, health-care management engineers are frequently in direct competition with external consultants. As many management engineers will admit, recommendations generated by outside consultants are often taken far more seriously than those proposed by in-house management engineers.

Conflicting and unclear roles. Management engineers have a widely divergent range of problem-solving tools at their disposal, and they seek to apply those tools to a wide variety of tasks from cost analysis to facility design. Many times, this role is in direct conflict with the roles performed by business school graduates, system analysts, accountants, computer scientists, and health-care economists.

During the past decade for example, more management engineers in the health-care field have become vice presidents, CEOs, or held other supervisory positions. It has been suggested that this is due partly to the limited scope of "functional staff." Until recently systems analysis, for example, was not considered to be one of the main thrusts of industrial engineering; yet there are many management engineers in the health-care field who end up working as systems analysts.

New nursing initiatives. The introduction of DRGs has compelled nursing to prepare itself for managing all patient care resources rather than only the clinical and supervisory functions. Today, more and more nursing school graduates are demonstrating a great deal of interest in areas such as cost analysis and fiscal management. Nursing is actively taking a leadership role in the areas of nursing care costs, quality assurance, and nursing productivity measurement. Even traditional IE areas, such as work sampling, have become a priority in the nursing field.

Also, some research has been done by the nursing profession on job stress, job design, job enlargement, decision-making, autonomy, and the like, and these are areas in which industrial engineers have often demonstrated some leadership.

As DRGs become a way of life in the health-care industry, one can expect rapid expansion in current research initiatives in nursing and the allied professions.

New needs. While the old needs of the health-care industry remain very important, management engineers in today's hospitals must probe for an effective balance between quality of patient care and the need for cost containment. Management engineers must take the lead in dispelling the notion that improved quality means higher costs and lower productivity.

With the introduction of DRGs, there now exists the need to move management engineering into an effective role of becoming "client centered." As a primary goal, management engineers must now address the question of how resource allocation in a fiscally constrained environment can result in more effective health-care delivery. The present health-care environment does not necessarily require new problem-solving tools, but rather a new perspective for the old tools. A summary of management engineering problem-solving tools and the differences between the old and new perspectives on the role of management engineers is presented in Table 10-1.

Table 10-1. Traditional versus new perspectives for hospital management engineers.

Factors	Traditional Perspectives	New Perspectives
1. Costs	Emphasis is on cost reduction; quality is expected to just happen.	Emphasis should be on quality of care, with primary focus on the patient.
2. Project focus	Focus is on enhancing profitability and the bottom line.	Projects should be client centered and quality-driven.
3. Productivity	Productivity is increased when services or resource use is reduced.	To increase productivity, quality should be continually improved.
4. Competition	Little attention is paid to the competition.	Greater attention should be paid to the competition.
5. Management's role	Management assumes that it knows best what the customer's quality requirements are.	Management should assume that the customer knows better and must be consulted through market research.
6. Definition of quality	Quality is defined according to JCAHO requirements.	Quality should be defined by customer's experience and expectations.
7. Quality assurance	Quality assurance is seen as a department function (managed through the QA department).	Quality assurance should be seen as everybody's responsibility, from secretaries to physicians.
8. Problem-solving	Problem-solving is localized within the management engineering group.	A multidisciplinary approach to problem-solving should be adopted through the use of QC teams, policy department, and quality in routine activities.
9. Problem-solving tools	Emphasis is on use of operations research tools, such as linear programming, simulation, queuing, etc. These tools are applied to arbitrarily selected problems.	Emphasis should be on the use of QC and operations research tools for solving highly prioritized, quality-oriented problems which directly impact the customer.
10. The customer	The patient is the customer.	A broader definition of the customer should be adopted: customers are patients, physicians, third party payers, patients' families and friends.

THE ROLE OF MANAGEMENT ENGINEERS IN THE QUALITY REVOLUTION

An understanding of the connection between quality and productivity is critical to managing quality in health care. The myth exists that if quality goes up, then costs go up and subsequently productivity decreases. Hospital management engineers, by virtue of their training and background, understand the correct nature of the relationship. They possess a reasonable understanding of the intervening variables linking productivity to quality and so can serve as facilitators in educating others in the health-care business. Management engineers understand that poor quality results in additional labor hours needed for correcting mistakes and wasted materials and supplies. The consequences of such inefficiencies are decreases in productivity, revenues, and profits. One of the challenges that management engineers face today is convincing health-care executives that continuous quality improvement leads to higher productivity.

Facilitators of Statistical Tools in TQM

Most leading experts in quality improvement agree on the importance of statistics in the quality management. It is important to understand the different types of statistical studies when conducting research for improving the quality of design, conformance, and performance, so that the information generated by the study can be used rationally as a basis for quality improvement action. Although there is evidence of limited use of statistics in hospitals, its use in the continuous improvement and monitoring of quality is only now gaining acceptance. This is due in part to the fact that the majority of hospital employees (clinical and non-clinical staff) have a limited (if any) background in statistics. Generally speaking, physicians, nurses, administrators, and the like often demonstrate a built-in fear of statistics and would resist any effort that makes statistics a part of their routine activities. Management engineers can use their strong analytical skills to facilitate the application of statistical tools in the management and control of quality.

Training Programs

Education and training are truly the backbones of the success of QC teams. Each individual involved should receive training in team leadership and in using statistical tools to measure and standardize gains, since these skills are key components of a successful quality improvement program. The basic functions of management engineers bring them in constant contact with the various departments of a health-care organization. They are, therefore, well-suited to play the role of trainers for a quality-conscious health-care organization. Management engineers can use their background in preparing educational materials for conducting training programs in all aspects of statistical quality control. They can train employees at all levels of the organization and keep abreast of new developments for training and application.

Data and Information Gathering

The types of data and information necessary to support a TQM program can be sometimes difficult to obtain. The role of management engineering as liaison between the computer information system and QC teams is very significant. The type, format, and quantity of information to be gathered must be carefully specified. A quality information system is defined by Juran and Gryna (1980) as an organized method of collecting, storing, analyzing, and reporting information on quality to assist decision makers at all levels. According to Juran and Gryna, the information needed by a quality information system includes:

- customer market research
- information on purchased parts and materials
- process data
- results of audits

Management engineers can assist in gathering data and other pertinent information required for quality improvement. Kivenko (1984) gives some key factors to be considered when developing a quality information collection system. Some of the factors are summarized below:

- clearly state purpose, functions, and system objectives
- involve all prospective users
- determine system input and output data requirements
- use visually appealing presentation forms
- provide summaries for management
- determine how often reports are needed and who needs them

If data is to be useful, it must be accurate and timely. Although no known attempt has been made to directly place a dollar value on useless data, it is believed that its cost must be tremendous. Management engineers can draw upon their analytical skills in determining the types, format, and reliability of desired data.

OPPORTUNITIES FOR CONTINUOUS IMPROVEMENT

The large amount of diversity in industrial engineering gives management engineers the opportunity to identify potential areas for improvement. Continuous improvement calls for doing the right things right. To accomplish that objective, management engineers must cover the full breadth of their field, from facility design/redesign to product management. Table 10-2 shows numerous areas of opportunities for continuous improvement.

EXERCISES

10-1. Conduct a study to determine what percentage of the projects undertaken by your hospital's management engineering staff is directly related to quality of care.

10-2. What is your hospital's perception of management engineers? If it is not favorable, discuss what factors are primarily responsible for its unfavorable status. How are management engineers perceived among nurses?

Table 10-2. Areas of opportunity for continuous improvement.

IE Activity	Applications
1. Facility Layout and Location	• Design and layout of nursing station, nursing units, optimum bed arrangements, radiology department, pharmacy, emergency rooms, etc. • Optimum location of a piece of expensive, non-movable equipment in a single facility. Optimum location for a blood bank, central supplies, pharmacy, or radiology, to service all other hospital departments. • Locating two or more new facilities at a time to serve existing facilities in the hospital. • Studying the impact on quality of care and architecture of different layout configurations.
2. Technology/ Information Management	• Conducting feasibility studies for adopting new technology. Establishing selection criteria. • Quality of care implications and information management of bedside terminals. • Software and hardware acquisition, selection, and evaluation. Comparison and analysis of various productivity, quality assurance, and patient classification software. • Analysis and implementation of bar coding in patient identification, prescriptions, accounting, etc. • Economic analysis of lease or buy decisions. • Developing productivity information data base to support a unit-based, client-centered, local productivity management program. Data base must include all resources used in patient care such as direct and indirect nursing care, ancillary costs, room and bed, overhead costs, etc., by patient, day, and DRG.
3. Work Measurement and Methods Improvement	• Conduct nursing workload measurements for staffing/patient classification system. • Establish time standards for highly routine and repetitive activities. E.g., admission, discharge, housekeeping. • Apply work sampling to direct and indirect nursing care, clerical work, major equipment use, operating rooms, outpatient waiting area, etc.
4. Human Factors/ Ergonomics and Safety	• Assess job stress among nurses; burnout factor among nurses. • Analyze lower back injury among nurses; problems with lifting, pushing, and pulling of patients. • Evaluate lighting, noise levels, temperature, and other environmental factors. • Consider design of work stations, beds, wheelchairs, surgical instruments, operating tables, and dental chairs.
5. Management Science/ IE/Operations Research Techniques	• Apply linear programming for studying menu planning, housekeeping, staffing, etc. • Apply forecasting techniques to areas of service demand, resource consumption, admissions, etc. • Apply simulation to study emergency rooms, operating rooms, admissions, discharge, resource utilization, X-ray labs, staffing, etc. • Apply queuing theory to transportation support services, labs, X-rays, operating rooms, emergency room, outpatient care, etc.

6. Quality Assurance and Control	• Validating and assessing various quality assurance instruments. • Developing quantitative indicators of quality care. • Using statistical control charts to monitor length of stay by DRG.
7. Human Resource Development	• Design and implementation of financial and nonfinancial incentive systems for particular groups within the health care field, e.g., DRG coders. • Study how employee turnover, absenteeism, and job satisfaction vary with age, experience, and qualification. • Job specialization, job evaluation, job rotation, job enlargement and job enrichment. • Study of recruitment and promotion philosophy from within or without. • Design and implementation of employee recognition programs. • Study of nurse-physician conflicts; RN-LPN conflicts and role assignment.
8. Organizational Management	• Central vs. decentral decision making. • Leadership characteristics of unit managers and goal realization. • Autonomy in decision making. • Management by objectives. Participative management concepts. • Decision latitude vs. job demand in nursing.
9. Productivity Management	• Analysis of outcome- vs. output-based measure of nursing productivity. • Nursing unit productivity measurement based on total resource consumption. • Diagnosis-based measure of productivity, profitability, and price recovery. • Partial productivity measures at the unit level. • Costing out of direct and indirect nursing services. • Developing cost breakdowns for all resources consumed in care delivery. • Studying the impact hospital policies have on unit productivity or resource consumption. • Developing a relationship between total productivity and quality of care. Developing a quality-adjusted total productivity model. • Development and implementation of a comprehensive unit-based total productivity management program. • Development of a "patient-centered" productivity measurement program for the various work centers.
10. Product Management	• Analysis of all 490 DRGs (or highest volume DRGs) for profitability, average length of stay, average resource consumption, price recovery, and seasonal and trend variations.

10-3. What percentage of your hospital's management engineers are presently performing functions not related to the traditional management engineering functions discussed in this chapter?

10-4. To what extent do your hospital's management engineers play the role of an integrator? Discuss implications for quality.

10-5. During the past five years, has there been any training program given by your hospital's management engineers? If so, for whom was the training designed?

BIBLIOGRAPHY

Bartscht, K. G. and R. Coffey. 1977. Management engineering — A method to improve productivity. *Topics in Health Care Financing*. Aspen Systems Corporation.

Covert, R. P. and E. McNulty. 1981. *Management Engineering for Hospitals*. Chicago, IL: American Hosptial Association.

DiVesta, N. 1984. The changing health care system: An overview. *DRGs: Changes and Challenges*. Franklin A. Shaffer, ed. New York: National League for Nursing. Pub. no. 20-1959.

Georgopoulos, B. R., ed. 1972. *Organization Research on Health Institutions*. Ann Arbor, MI: Institute for Social Research, University of Michigan.

Goldberg, Alan J. and Robert A. DeNoble, eds. 1986. *Hospital Departmental Profiles*, Second Edition. Chicago, IL: American Hospital Association (AHA).

Gray, S. P. and W. Steffy. 1983. *Hospital Cost Containment Through Productivity Management*. New York: Van Nostrand Reinhold.

Juran, M. M. and Gryna, Jr. *Quality Planning and Analysis*, 2nd ed. New York: McGraw-Hill.

Kivenko, K. 1984. *Quality Control for Management*. Englewood Cliffs, NJ: Prentice-Hall.

Nanda, R. 1986. Redesigning work systems — A new role for IE. *Fall Industrial Engineering Conference Proceedings*. Norcross, GA: Institute of Industrial Engineers.

Numerof, R. E. 1982. *The Practice of Management for Health Care Professionals*. New York: AMACOM.

Omachonu, V. K. and R. Nanda. 1988. A conceptual framework for hosptial nursing unit productivity measurement. *Industrial Engineering*. Norcross, GA: Institute of Industrial Engineers. 20(5):56.

_____. 1988. A diagnosis-based approach to hospital nursing unit productivity measurement. *Proceedings, 9th Annual Conference*. Knoxville, TN: American Society for Engineering Management.

_____. 1988. Hospital information and technology management under the prospective pricing system. *Proceedings of the First International Conference on Technology Management*. T. M. Khalil, et al., eds. Switzerland: Inderscience Enterprises Ltd.

_____. 1988. Developing a new data base for hosptial productivity information management. *Proeedings of the 10th Annual Computers and Industrial Engineering Conference*. Dallas, TX. 15:277.

_____. 1988. IEs in health care management must emphasize client-centered projects which contain cost while supporting quality. *Industrial Engineering*. 20(10):66.

Shaffer, Franklin. 1984. *DRGs: Changes and Challenges*. National League for Nursing. Pub. no. 20-1959.

Smalley, H. E. 1982. *Hospital Management Engineering*. Englewood Cliffs, NJ: Prentice-Hall International Series in Industrial and Systems Engineering.

Ziegenfuss, Jr., J. T. 1985. *DRGs and Hospital Impact*. New York: McGraw-Hill.

About the Author

Vincent K. Omachonu, Ph.D., P.E. is an assistant professor in the department of industrial engineering at the University of Miami, Coral Gables, Florida, and an adjunct professor in the Health Administration program, University of Miami School of Business. He has worked as a management engineer at Jackson Memorial Hospital, Miami, and has consulted for a variety of organizations including Baxter Healthcare Corporation and Ciba Geigy Corporation. He has published articles in technical and professional journals including *Health Care Management Review, Nursing Management,* and *Health and Human Resources Administration.*

Dr. Omachonu is a recipient of numerous teaching awards including the University of Miami (Freshman) Teaching Award and the School of Business Teaching Excellence Award. He has conducted numerous seminars on TQM for various organizations including IDAB Corporation and Broward General Hospital. Dr. Omachonu is a senior member of IIE, a member of ASQC, AHA, HSRA, and the University of Miami Institute for the Study of Quality.

Index

A t or f in parentheses indicates a table or figure.